MY DISABILITY IS DIVINE

"Amy Kenny has done it again. With humor, wit, and a vibrant depth of disability wisdom, Kenny invites us to recognize all the ways the disability community enriches our collective flourishing. This book is a celebration of life in all its forms, encouraging us to see disability as a fierce teacher of imagination, creativity, and ultimately divinity. Anyone seeking to expand their understanding of what it means to be human in our fullest, most radiant capacity needs to read this book."

—**Kat Armas**, theologian and author of *Abuelita Faith* and *Liturgies for Resisting Empire*

"Reading books about ableism and disability from disabled authors is one of the most important things we can do in our world today. Disability works as a moral, political, social, and spiritual compass, showing us who we are and directing us to where we should go, and Amy Kenny approaches this topic with great wit and deep wisdom. This book is a call, not just for the church but for all of us, to understand what got us here—the dehumanization and hatred contained in our explicit and implicit ableism—and to ask how we can move forward by honoring the stories and experiences of disabled folks while bearing witness to the prophetic voices they carry into the world that awaits us."

—**Kaitlin B. Curtice**, award-winning author of *Native and Everything Is a Story*

"*My Disability Is Divine* is a bold, visionary book that encourages readers to engage in a more profound and truthful discussion of disability and faith. Through personal narrative and theological reflection, Kenny exposes the ways ableism has shaped our spiritual imagination and calls us toward something more beautiful, more just, and more true. This book is deeply pastoral, offering hope to those who have been marginalized or misunderstood within faith communities. It's a courageous and compelling contribution to the disability justice movement, one that will challenge, comfort, and reshape how we understand both disability and the divine."

—**Lamar Hardwick**, author, scholar, and disability advocate

MY DISABILITY IS DIVINE

A Joyful Witness That Defies Ableist Nonsense

AMY KENNY

BrazosPress
a division of Baker Publishing Group
Grand Rapids, Michigan

Published by Brazos Press
a division of Baker Publishing Group
Grand Rapids, Michigan
BrazosPress.com

Printed in the United States of America

Library of Congress Cataloging-in-Publication Data
Names: Kenny, Amy, 1987– author
Title: My disability is divine : a joyful witness that defies ableist nonsense / Amy Kenny.
Description: Grand Rapids, Michigan : Brazos Press, a division of Baker Publishing Group, [2026]
Identifiers: LCCN 2026013577 | ISBN 9781587437045 paperback | ISBN 9781493456468 ebook
Subjects: LCSH: Disabilities—Religious aspects—Christianity | People with disabilities—Religious life
Classification: LCC BT732 .K36 2026
LC record available at https://lccn.loc.gov/2026013577

Some names and details have been changed to protect the privacy of the individuals involved.

Baker Publishing Group publications use paper produced from sustainable forestry practices and postconsumer waste whenever possible.

26 27 28 29 30 31 32 7 6 5 4 3 2 1

For every disabled person
who has the courage to imagine a world
where we can co-flourish.
May we never doubt that we are divine.

CONTENTS

PREFACE

We are made of the same stuff as stars. This is not merely a poetic image. The potassium in our muscle spasms, the carbon in our "overactive" nerves, the magnesium our chronically ill immune systems preserve, and the calcium in our curved spines are all made of the same stuff as the stars that shine. The bodyminds of disabled people[1] are made in the image of a God who knows the stars by name and delights in each of us as good—very good (Gen. 1:31; Ps. 147:4). Anything else would be a falsehood. We don't need to reach for the stars when their stardust has been within us all along. Our very worth is engraved in the galaxy.

Disability is divine. I am not merely starry-eyed when I say this. We are out of this world. Our crutches and bedazzled canes, our

1. Much ink has been spilled on whether we should use people-first language ("people with disabilities") or identity-first language ("disabled people") when talking about disability. I respect the various ways disabled people wish to be identified. Throughout the book, I typically use "disabled people." For me, choosing this language is a way of shunning the shame often associated with disability and proclaiming that "disability" is not a bad word or something to avoid. Disability is a part of the biodiversity of humanity, so I talk about it in a similar way to other aspects of my identity and experience.

push pops and neurodivergent brains, our sign names and wide doorframes, our access check-ins and stims, our rooms without fumes but plenty of spoons. Disabled people radiate the divine to an unsuspecting world with the way we sign, stroll, spin, stim, and shine.

This book is an invitation to consider the ways we are already benefiting from the wisdom and joy of our radiant disability community. I hope we can imagine a new world, where all of us can flourish. But disability is not all laughs and gaffes. Our lives contain ample grief, relief, and disbelief. Disability is a complex identity, full of delight and full of despair. So it seems only fitting for this book to orbit all of it: the giggles, the grime, the gore, and more. All of these experiences and emotions are present in our lives and are part of the way we understand ourselves, one another, and the divine.

On these pages, you will find pieces of my story that are tender to share and, perhaps, heavy to read. I hope you are well cared for as you let them wash over you. Broadly speaking, the book takes us on a journey of sorrow and joy, anger and adaptability, and seclusion and community. Disability is a broad constellation of experience. I am not the spokesperson or scapegoat for the entire community, nor do I want to be. This story is my own.

Disability is not linear or a monolith. One way this book wants to honor the complexity of disability is by matching form and feature. That means you are invited to engage with the pages in a variety of ways, reflection, doodling, and practices among them. I also want to care for you as the reader in giving you some loving spoiler alerts for what's to come.

How should you read this book? However you want! This book is written in a choose-your-own-adventure style. You can read the book straight through as it is written. Or you can choose a track that aligns with what you need in this moment.

Perhaps you're in a place where you don't need to read about medical stories right now. I got you. I've developed a track with you in mind. Perhaps you're in a place where you want to revel in art and radiance. Love this for you. There's a track with you in mind. Perhaps you need a playlist of the songs I reference in the book to get the vibe. I made it for us. You know I wouldn't play you like that. (Skip to the end of the book to scan the QR code to access the playlist.)

Choose your own adventure, then check out the chapters in this order:

- Art for art's sake: 1, 2, 6, 3, 9, 10
- Heartaches and heartbreaks: 4, 5, 6, 7, 9, 1
- No medical, for goodness' sake: 1, 2, 3, 5, 8, 9, 10, 11
- Joy you can't fake: 1, 2, 3, 5, 8, 9, 10, 11
- No nonsense, piece of cake: 1, 2, 3, 4, 5, 6, 7, 8, 9, 10, 11
- *Star Wars* hot takes: 4, 5, 6, 1, 2, 3, 7, 8, 9

May reading this book bring abundance and hope, especially in the moments that feel like we can no longer cope. May reading this book be an exhortation, an encouragement, and an ease. May reading this book remind each of us that we are already divine.

Shine bright, supernova.

1

MY DISABILITY IS DIVINE

It's not until the fifth person calls me "blasphemous" that I put down my phone. It turns out people don't like it when I describe my experience of God as disabled. A sound bite of a podcast where I talk about my experience of God quickly amassed more than fifty thousand views, more traffic than a California freeway at rush hour. Never mind that Scripture tells us in Daniel and Ezekiel that God's throne is a chair with wheels (ahem, wheelchair), or that the Spirit uses nonspeaking communication, or that I was simply sharing my experience of the divine.[1]

"Dr. Dummy," "blasphemous," "heretic," "a danger to the church," they branded me. "Jesus's resurrection isn't about you," another sneered, along with a bunch of ableist slurs for emphasis, just in case I missed the vibe. "F—— Amy Kenny for wanting attention" was uninspired but effective. Leviticus was quoted more

1. For more, check out Nancy L. Eiesland, *The Disabled God: Toward a Liberatory Theology of Disability* (Abingdon, 1994).

than once. But my favorite takedown was calling my reading of Scripture "narci-gesis," which even I had to admit was a clever pun.

My phone plummeted from my grip, but the messages still doomscrolled in my mind. The ableist slurs, the mocking memes, the jabs and jokes—all at my expense. All from Christians. It seems it's always from Christians. I tell myself the japes aren't about me, but I am the one who feels jilted by them all the same.

People advise me to have a thicker skin, to not let it affect me, to brush it off. That this treatment is expected when you publish a book or an opinion online and you are a disabled woman. That this is just part of The Discourse™. But why should my skin be thick because someone else's tolerance is so thin? Why is thick skin required to interact with people who should be known for our love? Why have we accepted this level of loathing declared in Jesus's name?

"Jesus wept" is all I can think to say.

It wasn't *just* Jesus who was weeping. Salty tears catch in the back of my throat as I remind myself that I have been called ableist slurs before and I will again. I have been blamed, shamed, and framed all because I'm disabled. Thick skin is my middle name. It is both painful and predictable.

I wish I could brush it off and say that I am above the fray, that I have numbed myself enough to not let it get to me; but the truth is, it hurts. It stings like salt in a wound. Somehow, I don't think this is what Jesus meant when urging us to stay salty (Matt. 5:13).

I pick up the debris of my dignity and drill myself to show grace. "Just keep swimming" becomes my mantra to get through it. To love anyway. To be the change I want to see. But some days I just want to yell, to raise hell, to tell them to get lost. I, too, have read Leviticus and am not afraid to use it (chapter 19, verse 14, to be exact).

I don't know how to love my online neighbors well when hate is expected, even encouraged. I don't know how to form thin places of connection with the divine when we are discipled to build up a thick skin. I don't know how to be human in an inhumane world.

Sometimes the haters quote Scripture at me. Leviticus, John 9, and Psalm 139 are the most frequent fliers to gotcha-ville. They baptize their ableism in Scripture and call it holy.[2]

Everyone wants to bust out Psalm 139 about God knitting us together in the womb—until who God knits is someone disabled. Then, somehow, I represent the "decay of humankind." (That's actually been said to my face IRL. Wonder what they say behind my back.) Somehow, Scripture is a takedown tool. It's as if it's Basic Instructions for Belittling Loathsome Enemies. The B-I-B-L-E, yes, that's the social media takedown for me.

It's in person too. People are quick to tell me that social media is the problem and that people are not as cruel to one another in person. Um, have they met people? Proximity, that's how we'll solve this puzzle, I've been lectured on repeat.

When people praise the power of proximity, I think about the friend I had dinner with every week who told me—not as a confession or lament but as an excuse—that disabled people messed up God's perfect plans. "Messed up" were the words he used, to my face, like I'm a supervillain who just succumbed to the dark side. Mwah ha ha ha ha ha. I wasn't the one letting the hate flow through you.

I think about the friend who claimed to "get it" because his dad was disabled, only to blame the Bible for his bias when it came time to support disabled people by buying a temporary ramp for our church. That's not stewarding tithe well, he enlightened me.

2. A working definition of "ableism": "A system of assigning value to people's bodies and minds based on societally constructed ideas of normalcy, productivity, desirability, intelligence, excellence, and fitness. These constructed ideas are deeply rooted in eugenics, anti-Blackness, misogyny, colonialism, imperialism, and capitalism." Talila A. Lewis, developed in community with disabled Black/Indigenous and negatively racialized people, "Working Definition of Ableism—January 2022 Update," January 1, 2022, https://www.talilalewis.com/blog/working-definition-of-ableism-january-2022-update.

I think about the churchgoer who somehow proclaimed "God doesn't make mistakes" while actively wishing her brother was not intellectually disabled, as though erasing who God made isn't blasphemy.

I think about the pastor friend who witnessed a fellow churchgoer shout at me through gritted teeth and reddening cheeks that we shouldn't care about disabled people, because that's not the gospel. My friend stayed silent, eyes glued to the floor, because, well, "good and godly people disagree."

I think about the friend who told me I need to be "less sensitive" when it came to a woman forcefully holding me down to pray me away after I asked her not to, because she was "just trying to be faithful." Imagine my surprise when I came to find out that *I* was actually the offender. My crime? Causing division by calling out this ableism in our church.

After I pointed out that grabbing someone without their consent is actually called assault, our pastor defended this behavior through, you guessed it, the intent loophole. "That wasn't how she *meant* it! She wasn't *trying* to be ableist by getting rid of disabled people." Um, okay? Her nail marks on my arm don't care about her intent. Plus, I was soon to learn that I need to not "give the devil a foothold in our community." Evidently, my mere existence has the power to conjure the Accuser himself. Not today, Satan.

All of these friends shared meals after hospital stays and during holidays and were part of life groups and life's loops. We went through everything together, from babies to baptisms to burials. But when it came down to it, *I* was the problem for pointing out that ableism was the problem, not the ableism itself. The devil is in the details.

Proximity proves nothing. One in four people in the US are disabled,[3] yet somehow, ableist language, laws, and systems are

3. Centers for Disease Control and Prevention, "Disability Impacts All of Us," April 14, 2025, https://www.cdc.gov/disability-and-health/articles-documents/disability-impacts-all-of-us-infographic.html.

more rampant than ramps.[4] The math just doesn't add up. If proximity in and of itself were so powerful, we would witness an end to this ableist nonsense in our churches and communities. Where are the receipts?

Proximity works only if people are willing to change, and in my experience, many nondisabled Christians are unwilling to change because they think nothing is wrong with the way things are. Because they have been taught to use the Bible as a bullet for bigotry instead of a leader in love. Because they do not think of us as fully human.

But God does. God takes credit for us, disabilities and all. When Moses tries to get out of advocating to Pharaoh because of his speech disability, God claps back, "Who gives speech to mortals? Who makes them mute or deaf, seeing or blind? Is it not I, the LORD? Now go, and I will be with your mouth and teach you what you are to speak" (Exod. 4:11–12).

Moses is at peak "New phone, who dis?" He tries to dodge the invite, but God doesn't let him get away with it. God provides a divine accommodation for Moses in the form of Aaron. There is no talk of cure or condemnation; no concept that a disability could prevent Moses from advocating on God's behalf for enslaved people, no accusation of disrupting the unity. In fact, the notion that Moses's disability would be a deterrent is preposterous to God.[5] God is having none of it.

God calls Moses out and tells him the truth: God made disabled people and claims us, disabilities and all. There's no need for divine

4. I don't represent all disabled people, of course. This book is written from my experience. "Disability" is a big word with a lot of meanings. There are long histories of how this word has been and still is weaponized. Not everyone with what we might call disability experience identifies as disabled, nor do they need to. For many, identifying as disabled can be dangerous. I am not the gatekeeper of who is part of the community. For more on disability identity, check out Sami Schalk, *Black Disability Politics* (Duke University Press 2022), 132.

5. For more on Moses, check out Julia Watts Belser, *Loving Our Own Bones: Disability Wisdom and the Spiritual Subversiveness of Knowing Ourselves Whole* (Beacon, 2023), 74.

intervention in the form of erasing or excluding disability, because God is proud of making disabled people just the way we are.

The next time a stranger approaches a disabled person with "No Wheelchairs in Heaven" (an actual poem I've received in the last month) or the evergreen "What sin is preventing you from walking?" I want us to clap back by quoting God: *Who* made disabled people? Is it not God?

Disability is not a flaw but a fabulous feature. And one that the creator of the universe takes credit for. It's weird for people who claim to have a "biblical worldview" to not take God seriously in this passage. Narci-gesis, anyone?

If connecting my disabled bodymind to God bothers other people, that seems like an other-people problem. Or, to quote Lamar Hardwick, a.k.a. the Autism Pastor, "We are so ableist that we even discriminate against God."[6] God doesn't just tolerate our disabilities; God takes credit for them. God wants us to be a part of the community whether Christians do or not. God recognizes that disabled people are divine.

This book is about how disability is divine. To be divine is to be of, from, or like God.[7] Being divine doesn't mean we are not human or that we are removed from all the gunk, guts, and gore of humanity. It means that we are of, from, or like God. When I think about being *of* something, I picture identity, belonging, and constitution. *Of* can share where someone is from, who someone's family is, or who someone hopes to be (Francis *of* Assisi, Joan *of* Arc, and Juana Inés *de* la Cruz). *Of* can signal something's origin story (fruit *of* the Spirit or Fruit *of* the Loom). *Of* can state what something is made from (house

6. Lamar Hardwick, *How Ableism Fuels Racism: Dismantling the Hierarchy of Bodies in the Church* (Brazos, 2024), 115.

7. *Oxford English Dictionary*, accessed September 27, 2025, under "divine," https://www.oed.com/dictionary/divine_adj.

of cards or abs *of* steel). When I say we are divine, I mean we are *of* God.

We know that humans were made in the likeness of God (Gen. 1:26; 5:1–3). We reflect God's image right here, right now. There is nothing we can do or say that can take that away. When I say we are divine, I mean we are created in God's likeness.

Saying we are divine doesn't mean that we have supernaturally transcended being human. We are not spooks, specters, or sprites. We are not gremlins or genies. We are not K-pop demon hunters (but we are golden). Nor do I endorse this statement to spiritually bypass the grim realities of our lives. That can be really harmful. Saying we are divine is a core belief that each one of us is fully, inherently, unequivocally of, from, or like God.

Many of us have been led to believe that disabled people are some sloppy seconds, a group of wayward wannabes, when nothing could be further from the truth. Disabled people reflect God's image. Disabled people are created in the likeness of God. Disabled people share in God's holiness.[8] To put it simply, disabled people are divine.

This is what I wish people knew when they called me blasphemous for daring to talk about my experiences with God. Instead, they are quick to call me names I don't feel comfortable repeating, all in Jesus's name.

I am many things. I am a disabled white woman with apparent and nonapparent disabilities who uses a variety of mobility aides to move about the world. I am a daughter, sister, spouse, auntie, coconspirator, confidant, and fierce friend. I am the descendant of convicts who worked the land that is now known as Australia, land that was already home to the Gadigal people of the Eora Nation. I am Australian by birth, American by migration, and of a third culture that is both and neither of these tapestries of experience. I am not a parent but have been proudly dubbed "mother." I hope

8. For more on these concepts, check out Eph. 4:24, Heb. 12:10, and 2 Pet. 1:4.

I am a good ancestor, co-creating new ways of flourishing for all who follow. I am a scholar, an educator, and a learner. I hate small talk but love big ideas. I am more at home in the water than on land. I snort when I laugh, and I've never met a pie I didn't like. Jalapeños are my love language. I am many things, but ableist slurs are not who I am. In fact, it is the ableism that is blasphemous.

I have a well-developed grace muscle for this ableist nonsense. I know how to spot a wolf in sheep's clothing, and I know that this does not smell like Jesus. Yet I wish I did not need such a muscle, or that I was not used to this maelstrom of mistreatment from people who call themselves my siblings in Christ. I wish church folks were more interested in loving than loathing.

The most popular question I get asked in response to sharing my story is, "Which denomination are you a part of?" This comes with a scrumptious side of assurances that praying away disabled people wouldn't happen in *their* church. People want to know what denomination did that horrible ableist thing to me so they can distance themselves.

This is not a denominational problem. I have been a part of megachurches and home churches, churches with an AV budget bigger than my annual salary, and churches without heat. I've been a part of churches that meet in old sanctuaries, new warehouses, decorated living rooms, dilapidated classrooms, or Zoom rooms. We've sat in crimson velvet pews, flip-up theater seats, and camping chairs. I've been a part of churches with a long list of "what we believe" on the website, and ones without a website at all. The Lord's table has spanned from a matzo cracker to stale bread to a banquet, accompanied by everything from wine on a silver platter to a plastic juice thimble with a tear-off lid.

I've been a part of churches where my fellow churchgoers wave American flags, Pride flags, Christian flags, Don't Tread on Me flags, Thin Blue Line flags, and Black Lives Matter flags. Bells and smells? Check. Nondenominational? To name a few. When it comes to churches, I've been there, done that, got the HE>i sticker. This is not a denominational problem.

I have been a part of many church communities in my life, with different dogmas and doctrine, size and scale, locations and liturgies, but they all have one thing in common: None of them have publicly disabled[9] pastors, elders, or preachers.

None of them talk about disability theology or the ways we learn from the leadership and wisdom of the disability community. And *all* of them have preached and practiced ableism.

So before we distance ourselves and our denominations from the ableism that so frequently festers unchecked in our churches, let's ask ourselves: How many of our pastors, priests, leaders, teachers, sisters, elders, or counselors are disabled? How many people are disabled in your inner circle whom you seek guidance from? How many disabled people in your community would count you as a trusted friend?

I hope you prove me wrong.

"I have a confession to make," he blurts out. I hold my breath as the words spill out of his mouth, my lungs wrung out at the word "confession."

"I *want* to include disabled people," he claims, "but the truth is, I just can't picture a *good* God allowing disabled people into heaven. Disabled people aren't God's plans for perfection."

Breathe, I coach myself internally as I count. If I make it to ten, I know I can cut down on the finger-wagging tone of my voice.

I get to nine before noticing him open his mouth again, so I blurt out, "If you can't picture disabled people in heaven, then I

9. "Publicly disabled" in this context refers to people who publicly disclose their disability, including apparent, nonapparent, and dynamic disabilities.

guess Jesus can't be there." I yank up the speed of my wheels from tortoise to hare and hop away before he can respond.

Ever since my book *My Body Is Not a Prayer Request* came out, I've become a confessional. People want to confess all of their ableism to me, as if admitting it will make it go away. They haven't done the work; they haven't changed their ways; they want to skip ahead to the finish line. They want a participation trophy engraved with "Disability Ally."

They want absolution, not justice.

Like the pastor who admitted, without repentance, that she prayed for wheelchair users to have more faith and walk, adding, "That's what I was trained to do in seminary," as if that makes it any better.

Or the church elder who reflected to me, with no signs of blushing, that he hadn't realized disabled people even had opinions about God before reading my book. They didn't know we were capable of faith. Surprise, we are people too!

Or the group who disclosed that their church isn't accessible, not because they don't care but because of budget. Accessibility costs money, and only helps *some* people, but donuts and coffee are for everyone, so they can't cut *that* budget. I understand that, right? Oh, I understand perfectly. Camel, meet eye of needle.

It turns out I am everyone's one disabled friend, accepting their casual confessions about all the ableism they never knew they had. They want to be coddled into believing that they are *different* from the church folks who fought against the Americans with Disabilities Act (ADA). They want to be told they are a good person and it's okay that they didn't know that in the United States, disabled people *still* don't have (1) marriage equality, (2) minimum wage protections, or (3) access to religious communities.

But the truth is, it's not okay. It's not okay to demand our gratitude for doing the bare minimum of learning what ableism is.

It's not okay if the way you gather excludes us.

It's not okay to heap the emotional labor on me, as if *I* should thank you for realizing that disabled people are, in fact, people. We are 16 percent of the global population and 28 percent of the US population.[10] If we can't understand that one-fourth of our neighbors are fully human, then we might have lost the plot of church a long time ago.

People think they are doing something extra when they treat us as human beings. They want us to be grateful just because we can get into the building or because they suddenly realize folks communicate in diverse ways. Or because there's a place for (some of) us to pee. Ableism keeps us grateful.

I want to tell casual confessionals all this. I want to tell them the pain of being dissed, dismissed, forgotten, or forced into performing gratitude. I want to tell them Matthew 25 from the ASV, the Amy Standard Version:

> Depart from me, for I used a wheelchair, and you gave me no ramp. I tried to get in the front door, and you said it costs too much money. I just wanted to be a part of the beloved community, and you said, "Disabled people don't belong here." Whatever you did for disabled people, you did for me.

But I don't always tell them this, because I don't think it smells like Jesus for me to tell strangers that all the time. And because we need nondisabled people to understand our humanity. Our survival depends on it.

But I don't want to just survive; I want to thrive. I want to share the joys of our disability community. To revel in the ways that disability has added to all of our lives. I don't want to use the tools of ableism, white supremacy, xenophobia, queerphobia, and

10. "Disability," World Health Organization, March 7, 2023, https://www.who.int/news-room/fact-sheets/detail/disability-and-health; Centers for Disease Control and Prevention, "Disability Impacts All of Us."

misogyny to construct our own exclusive community. I want us to dismantle them all together.

I don't want absolution, I want justice.

I want community. Not a community centered on who we are against, as if the only thing we have in common is that we hate the same people. Common enemy intimacy is not community.[11] Not a community where we all compete for gold in the Oppression Olympics. None of us medal that way. I want us to recognize the divinity in one another. I want us to learn from the disability wisdom of creation what it means to co-flourish.

In fact, it was the trees that whispered my worth long before any church community did. *Crooked*, the white coats had told me on repeat. My leg is crooked. My alignment is "off." But little in nature is straight; creation is charmingly crooked. The bent branches of the bonsai, the meandering roots of the mangroves, the curls of the corkscrew willow. Creation is vibrantly crooked.

It is human-made stuff that is "orderly" and "logical." But the canvas of creation is wild, unruly, and exquisitely messy. Creator's invisible qualities are clearly witnessed throughout nature, and they are delightfully disabled (Rom. 1:20).[12]

Everywhere I turn, I marvel at nature displaying radiant disability. Crooked bushes—real name—are hunched, sprawling their limbs outward in every which direction. Their branches are like my "crooked" body, bent and beautiful in our distinctiveness.

The hues of crimson and carrot that sweep across the autumn trees are due to cold temperatures, shorter days, and less

11. For more on common enemy intimacy, check out Brené Brown, *Braving the Wilderness: The Quest for True Belonging and the Courage to Stand Alone* (Random House, 2017), 135–36.

12. Throughout the book, I often use "Creator" to refer to God, following the wisdom of the First Nations Version translation of the New Testament, and to expand our understanding of the divine. For more, check out *First Nations Version: An Indigenous Translation of the New Testament* (InterVarsity, 2021).

chlorophyll. The vibrant color change we witness signals the *lack* of productivity of these trees. We might say that the trees are following their access needs, resting instead of producing. This sounds a lot like spoonie and disability wisdom to me.[13]

We can't always produce—we don't always have the energy to hustle—and just like the trees, we are vibrant and worthy of care. People mock us for knowing our limits, but we know the disability wisdom of following the rhythms of rest.

Deep beneath the ocean's surface, an octopus has arms growing out of its head and can camouflage to hide from predators. These masters of disguise change their tint and texture to replicate nearby rocks and coral. Their physiological changes are much like the fluidity of dynamic disability, which describes the experience of access needs fluctuating from day to day. Some days I need help getting dressed and some days I don't, but *all* days I can knock your socks off. And on all days, I am worthy of belonging and care.

No one claims kangaroos are feeble because they cannot walk backward. No one mocks sharks for communicating without speaking. The sound effect we associate with "shark!" is courtesy of *Jaws*, not nature. The ostrich is not weaker than the oriole because it cannot fly. We do not dismiss armadillos because they are hard of hearing, or elephants because they are born blind. No one claims lions have chronic fatigue syndrome because they languish almost all hours of the day. They are fast and fierce! They just act more like us spoonies than workaholics.

It turns out that the community of creation is disabled. The jaggedly majestic branches of the Japanese maple, the blind star-nosed mole, the flightless penguin. Nature is delightfully disabled. And so am I.

13. For more on spoon theory, check out Christine Miserandino, "The Spoon Theory," in *Beginning with Disability: A Primer*, ed. Lennard J. Davis (Routledge, 2017), 174–78.

Throughout creation, we value the biodiversity that disability brings. Yet we've often failed to apply this value to humans.

What if we tried? What if we reconsidered the way we understand disability, so that disabled people are not just tolerated but celebrated? What if we recognized that we are better together? What if we understood my wheels as I do—an empowering throne that generates access and agency?

It was the community of creation that proclaimed my own radiance to me. I started to realize that if I could marvel at the vibrance of disability in creation, then why couldn't I believe it about myself?

I started to allow myself to wonder, *What if I, too, am divine?* If I could consider the lilies of the field and the birds of the air as radiant, how come I hadn't thought that about myself when confronted with a mirror, mirror, on the wall?

What if we fostered a community of care not based on everything that we are against but out of affirming the dignity and divinity of each one of us, just as we are? What if we recognized that disability is divine?

Perhaps if we expanded our imaginations to understand the vibrancy and vitality of disability, we could experience the divine presence in our disabled neighbors.

And then I started to realize that throughout Scripture, we encounter disabled people at the forefront of the relationships that Creator cultivates with humanity.[14] Isaac becomes blind. Jacob walks with a limp and uses a cane in the cloud of witnesses. Moses has a speech disability. Elijah tells us about his depression. Timothy is chronically ill. Zacchaeus is a little person. Many of

14. I realize that our modern notion of disability is not the same as the notion common in antiquity. Throughout the book, I am not anachronistically diagnosing anyone or ascribing an identity but inviting us to consider experiences we might now understand as disabled. For more on this nuance, check out Amos Yong, *Theology and Down Syndrome: Reimagining Disability in Late Modernity* (Baylor University Press, 2017).

our autistic siblings read Noah as neurodivergent. And who can forget about Paul's thorn in the flesh? Or that the Great Banquet is accessible?

Too often, we erase these disabilities when we talk about Scripture because they make nondisabled people uncomfortable. But make no mistake, disabled folks are part of our Scriptures and spiritual traditions. We are a vibrant, whole, radiant part of the beloved community, and we are divine.

We are not God, nor do we need to be. We are humans, and by virtue of being human, we emanate the image of God and partake in the divine nature (2 Pet. 1:4). There is no asterisk or caveat excluding disabled people from these divine dealings. Nor do we await an afterlife to be able to partake. We reflect the divine presence to an unsuspecting world, just as we are.

I started to wonder if Creator, too, could understand a life on wheels. And I found God there, in a passage in Daniel, sitting on a "throne of fiery flames, and its wheels burning fire" (7:9). A chair with wheels sounds a lot like a wheelchair to me.

And again, I found a disabled God, in Ezekiel, where God is a radiant fire with a massive mobility device, lifted up by four angels with fused legs and colossal wheels. These wheels encase wheels that glisten like topaz.

My wheels liberate me and grip the pavement, absorbing the shock waves my body would otherwise have to endure. I lean in as we go around the corner, like water caressing a riverbank as it flows. I feel the texture of the earth, the rhythm of the cement. I hear the symphony of vibrations as we drift from concrete to cobblestone. My physicality does not stop at the tip of my toes or the crown of my head but extends to the frame of my cobalt chair, able to transport me to new worlds. Just like Ezekiel's vision, I am fused with wheels that are my ticket to freedom. I am body, wheel, and fire.[15]

15. Amy Kenny, *My Body Is Not a Prayer Request: Disability Justice in the Church* (Brazos, 2022), 153.

My disabled bodymind is made in the image of God, and Creator's invisible qualities are witnessed in disabled nature. So it makes sense to me to understand God as disabled. God uses a glowing, fire-flowing wheelchair, and so shall I.

Being disabled isn't just a series of medical appointments, mobility devices, or can't-dos. Disability is a culture and an embodied experience that shifts over time and can teach nondisabled people what it means to be human. To me, disability is an expansive and generative way of being. Disability is apparent and nonapparent and everything in between. You don't have to identify as disabled to experience disability. Our bodyminds and access needs morph over time, much like what we experience of Creator in Scripture and in our lives.

God takes on forms outside the norm. God is a burning bush and a pillar of fire. God communicates in groans too deep to utter, outside of verbalized language. We might call the Spirit nonspeaking. Creator is the cloud that guides our way. God is in the soggy fleece, the fiery furnace, the whirlwind, the wisdom and warning of a dream, and the widow's empty jar. God can be found in the mouth of a donkey, in the great fish, the gentle lamb, the mother hen, and the descending dove. And if that's not enough, even the rocks will cry out!

Creator is thunderclap and living water. God is in the still, small voice and the shining stars above. God is not in a hurry and moves at the speed of love.

Creator transforms our understanding of divinity into places we don't expect. And to me, God is delightfully disabled. And so am I. Together we can form a community where we recognize the divinity of disability so we can all flourish.

You might not realize it, but you are probably already benefiting from disability culture. Everything from texting to the touch screen to the electric toothbrush was created by and for disabled folks.

The next time we use a potato peeler or put on a Snuggie, I want us to think about the ingenuity of the disabled people who designed them. The next time we participate in a team huddle, I want us to know that was devised by the Deaf Gallaudet football team, who didn't want the other team spying their signs. Now we all benefit from this Deaf gain.

The next time we think "disability," I want us to think "creativity." Disabled folks are uniquely creative, because we live in a world not built for our bodyminds. We are equipped with a divine creativity to solve problems that nondisabled people didn't even know we had. Disability is a creative force that invites us to dream up a new world.

Imagine what we could design together if we stopped thinking of disability as a loss and recognized it as a variety of experiences, including many gains. Imagine the world we could create together if we were united not by who we condemn but by who we champion. Imagine if we stopped demanding gratitude from one another for meeting basic access needs so we can roll, walk, stim, and sign our way to co-flourishing.

Maybe you, too, are wondering about your worth. Maybe you are wondering if you count, or if you are disabled "enough." I will not wait for the willows to whisper it to you. Let me be the one to tell you.

You are divine. You, with so few spoons, you don't give a fork. You, who want to believe, but you're not sure if you do anymore. You, who know how winsome words like "inspirational" and "articulate" can be weaponized. You, who feel too churchy for your activist friends and too activist-y for your church friends. You, who have had to fight for your identity to be respected.

You, who cringe at the words "God's throne," but deep down, you still want them to mean something. You, who have more stickers on your water bottle than zeros in your bank account.

You, who don't yet have a name for your pain but know it is real, despite what the disability doubters say. You, who are sick of performing gratitude for the bare minimum. You, who aren't sure where you belong. I am glad that you are here.

You are divine. No caveats. No cures. No condemnation. The whole community of creation declares your worth.

Just as you are, you are divine.

PRACTICE

Were there any stories from Scripture mentioned in this chapter that surprised you? Were there any connections with disability that gave you pause? A lot of unlearning our assumptions about disability happens by revisiting stories we thought we knew with a fresh perspective. We might find a new detail or realize something that we previously assumed.

What is a story in Scripture that portrays disabled people that you might want to reconsider? In your sanctified imagination, how might you revisit that story or portrayal of disability?

Choose a passage of Scripture or an image to use. Not sure where to start? Borrow one of mine: Exodus 4, John 9, or "Wheelchair Christ" or "Blind Christ" by Rachel Holdforth.*

- *Observe.* Read the passage or behold the image. What do you notice? Slow down there, speed racer! Take it in again. This time, try to take in each detail. Let the details wash over you like rain on dry soil.
- *Reflect.* What connected with you? What brings you joy? What feels sticky? What feels exciting? Challenging? Comforting? If you can, invite your reflections without judgment.
- *Respond.* What might the passage or image tell us about disability? How can we understand it in light of this chapter about disability as divine? If you can, try to approach with curiosity instead of certainty.
- *Rest.* Take a deep breath. Check out the passage or image again. Be still, and know that disabled people are divine.

* Rachel Holdforth, "Wheelchair Christ" and "Blind Christ," linoprints, https://www.wobblygoose.com/wheelchair-christ and https://www.wobblygoose.com/blind-christ.

2

MY DISABILITY IS INNOVATIVE

The first thing we witness the Almighty do is create. It seems so simple, but I have come to understand this as profound. The God we meet in Scripture is one whose first task is not about power, greed, or speed but creativity. God is an artist.

First it was the light. Creator separates the bright from the night and calls it good. All the while, I picture God singing, "I'm in the stars tonight / So watch me bring the fire and set the night alight." It's dynamite. Next comes the sky, the seas, and the land. Then the seeds, the trees, and the plants. I picture the trees sprouting forth from the ground, outstretching their crooked limbs and boasting their magnificence to all around. Here comes the sun, the moon, and the stars to govern the skies, but not before God marvels at each with pride.

By the time God delights in the seal, the eel, and the turtle too, creation is swimming with a chorus of crustaceans in the deep blue. Each of these aquatic animals is remarkable. God did it on porpoise. With each new creature, God admires them and affirms their inherent goodness by blessing them all—the crab, the clam, and the clownfish. This isn't merely clocking a checklist of creatures but crafting that comes with a side of sanctifying. It seems like God is having a whale of a time!

Enter the blue jay, the osprey, and the parakeet. I wonder, did the robin regale Creator with a symphony complete? Did the peacock parade its plumage to the beat? How long was it before the kookaburra kicked back and cackled with the Paraclete? (My money is on dawn or dusk, since that's when they laugh to bond with their fleet.)

Imagine the creativity needed to dream up the moose, the mongoose, the baboon, and the raccoon; to put into motion the iguana, the goanna, the pug, and the slug; to call forth the hare, the mare, and the polar bear.

Imagine coming up with an animal that can pack a punch as quick as a bullet; one with three stomachs and a fleece mullet; one that poops square; or a duck-billed, egg-laying, beaver-tailed mammal that glows green, if you dare. (A mantis shrimp, an alpaca, a wombat, and a platypus, in case you were wondering.) Imagine igniting the premise that a worm with legs could one day become a beautiful bug with wings. How else would we know how to float like a butterfly, sting like a bee?

Imagine encoding skin with spots, fur with stripes, feathers that shine like metal, and scales that glint like gems. God loves a metallic. Pink dolphins, red ants, orange tigers, yellow canaries, green sea turtles, blue poison dart frogs, indigo snakes, and violet honeycreepers. All the colors of the rainbow are the canvas of creation. Patterns, palates, and textures galore!

The community of creation includes claws, jaws, hooves, and hands. Wings, whiskers, and webbed feet, prehensile tails and the shell of a snail. The rock-climbing ibex has suction-cupped hooves and a reflective coat to protect from heat, while the ibis comes with enough bill-sensitivity to search for scraps to eat. (Now I feel kinda bad for calling them "bin chickens.") It is perhaps unremarkable to us now that the gangly giraffe struts its stuff or that the rattlesnake knows how to shake its groove thing. Our world is so full of marvelous biodiversity that we often fail to notice the magnitude and magnificence of it all.

And then there were humans. With every curve and nerve, humans shine Creator's image to the world. The creativity of figures and features is fabulous. All of the radiant hair textures, all of the resplendent complexions, undertones, and highlights, all of the luminescent limbs that twist, spasm, and spark. All of the marvelous variety in the way our brains process, assess, and express. The variation alone is incandescent. We woke up like this. Or the way God tells it: We are good. *Very* good. *You* are very good!

By the time humans enter the scene, it's been busy. God's been at it again, crafting and coding new creatures big and small, from the flea to the manatee. God needs a nap. Who doesn't?

I love that the story includes rest. God has to rest from all the creating (Gen. 2:3), which can be weary work. In Scripture, we don't witness an aloof god pumping out fast facsimiles on the factory floor with little feeling and maximum efficiency. God delights in each creation, celebrating that it is good, and then relishes in the resting. This is a God who is familiar with the delicate dragonfly and the robust rhinoceros. This is a God who is less concerned with power and productivity than with creativity. This is a God who makes clothing and cuisine. This is a God who stops, slows down, and sings our praises.

Many of us have been introduced to a distant sky daddy acting hot-tempered and cold-hearted, particularly when it comes to dealing with us humans. But the God we meet here in Scripture is more concerned with artistry than anger. The God we meet here is connected to creation through delight. The God we meet here is one who cares enough about human shame to clap back, "Who told you?" in the same tone as when a friend responds to a shame spiral with, "Don't talk about my friend like that!" The God we meet here values us, just as we are.

I have come to understand that many churchy folks who rail against my disabled bodymind have a complicated relationship with their own value and worth. Many have a hard time believing that they are good enough or are worthy of love and care. It is hard to love your neighbors as yourself when you have been taught to loathe yourself. I wish this were not the case. Not just for them, but for all of us. The creator of the universe marvels at us and declares us very good. If only we could believe it.

God invites us to share in the responsibility of tending, nourishing, and nurturing creation. We are invited to co-create as part of the way we live, love, and learn. We are not robots carrying out the will of another. Nor are we a military force without agency enforcing a cosmic agenda. Sorry, Stormtroopers. We are human, and as humans, we get to create. Creativity is an outflowing of the divine in and with us. Creativity is just one way we radiate the image of God into the world, because creativity is divine.

In the Scriptures, God is a potter, a storyteller, an artist, and an architect. God takes what was once a valley of dry bones and breathes new life into it. God is crafty. And what God makes isn't some cheap knockoff or a sleazy side hustle. God is a creator of masterpieces, bangers, and bops. And what God devises is so delightful, so radiant, so magnificent, that we are told over and over again how good it is. Because it is you. It is me. It's the community of creation.

Anytime we breathe life into the community of creation, we are co-creating. Anytime we draw, decoupage, dance, doodle, or dream, we are emulating God. It doesn't have to be "for" anyone or anything; it doesn't even have to be savvy or skilled. So, sing your heart out. Anytime we do the holy work of restoration, we are showcasing the divine presence. Restoring is not fixing or faking; it is transforming, imagining, creating. Every time we honor that our bodyminds need rest, we follow Creator.[1]

1. For more on the sacredness of rest, check out Tricia Hersey, *Rest Is Resistance: A Manifesto* (Little, Brown Spark, 2022).

This is true of all humans—sometimes it's just forgotten when it comes to our disability community. Creator has instilled in us a divine ingenuity to solve problems that many nondisabled people didn't even know we had. Disability is a creative force that invites us to reimagine the world as we know it. We are intuitively imaginative and innovative because the current world is not built for our bodyminds.

The generative work of disability is not related to productivity but to our presence in the world. It is not merely our creative problem-solving that makes us worthy of dignity and respect. No accolade or accomplishment can instill us with more worth than what we already have. Disabled people are worthy solely because we are divine. Yet our creativity is a cultural wealth that benefits everyone. Many of us are already using assistive technology designed by and for disabled people every time we check our phones or brush our teeth. Disabled people are already creating new pathways for the whole world to flourish.

So many of our ideas and innovations benefit the broader population. We are just the ones who are brave enough to dream up a different way for things to be. We are the ones who know the weight of going first. We are the canaries in the coal mine who sing loudly that something is wrong long before others seem to notice. Our disability cultural wealth is treasured whether society recognizes it or not.

Imagine the world we can build together when we do.

"Down here!" I say to the audience, trying to defuse the tension. I am giving a guest lecture, but not at the lectern. We had to switch venues after the first one wasn't wheelchair accessible. The exterior of this one is, but the podium is not. One piece of furniture and a lot of ignorance prevent me from the architectural respect most guest speakers take for granted.

Wobbly, I seesaw my notes on my lap since the podium is not accessible to me. Too high, too narrow, too immovable, the podium rests to my right while I engage the audience using jokes as my armor. If only the podium could fit me.

Halfway through the presentation on disability culture, it occurs to me: What if the podium *could* fit me? We have sit-to-stand desks, so why not have sit-to-stand podiums?

Afterward, I ask around to find such a thing and am met with little more than lost looks, but I don't let that stop me. Solution: Invite our graduate students to design a more accessible version. Before prototyping the podium, students learn about threshold concepts of universal design and the idea that all designs have end users, and many of those end users are disabled.[2]

We dream up how we can integrate sensory tools, braille, width adjustment, and of course, a sit-to-stand feature that can change the height of the podium with the push of a button. We even incorporate a battery pack to ensure the podium can adjust heights for different speakers throughout one event without connectivity to power.

We prototype with cardboard and Popsicle sticks. One design looks like a tripod martian with tentacles crawling up and down. One has duct-taped wings that flap like a pheasant. They are supposed to be for privacy, but they need some refinery. One has captions displayed on the front of the podium itself before being scrapped for lack of legibility. These scheme-and-dream sessions invite students to remix what they have previously known. We redesign what a podium could be through research, applied learning, prototyping, and dreaming. Or, to put it another way, we question why things are the way they are, and imagine how they could be better. Our accessible lecterns are held together by duct tape and dreams.

2. Many thanks to Sarah Craig, Michael Pasimio, Maggie Debelius, David Strout, and Yianna Vovides for their partnership on bringing this project to life.

The end result isn't just a podium but a paradigm shift. Many of the students shared with me that, before the class, they had never considered how a podium might not be accessible to everyone. It was fixed, a stationary element that had no cause for reinvention. But what if it could be flexible?

First came the shift. Students started to consider what else could be altered to allow for more people to flourish. Then came the stories about how the podium produced belonging we didn't initially anticipate. A four-foot-eight-inch-tall guest speaker who had previously brought a soapbox of sorts, cleverly concealed inside a podium, no longer needed a booster. A tall ballplayer who had to request a custom podium that would fit his height no longer needed to preorder access. A little person who previously schlepped his own pop-up tabletop apparatus to avoid the dehumanizing comments about his stature no longer needed to lug his own portable podium around. A staff member who no longer twinged their back in setting up the lectern, thanks to the wheels. Lecterns are not one-size-fits-all. What started as a life hack for wheelchair users expanded to a culture of access for a community. Having no lectern is a champagne problem, but what is sobering is how much access labor is required in every avenue of life. This is not a story about one lectern. This is a story about how we can redesign the way things are so that all of our bodyminds can thrive.

We call this the curb-cut effect, when something designed to meet access needs supports everyone, regardless of whether they identify as disabled. Curb cuts ease the path for parents with strollers crossing the street. They support techs with trolleys of audiovisual equipment and caterers with trays of yummy treats. They make the paths smooth for anyone with a suitcase, a dolly, a wagon, a bike, or a cart. Curb cuts offer access to much more than wheelchair users, yet they were designed by and for the disability community for everyone to thrive. Disabled people dream up interdependent ways of being together that benefit everyone. Our cultural wealth pays dividends for all to flourish.

One of the most frustrating parts about being disabled is that the nondisabled people who fight against creating a culture of access end up benefiting from it. Curb cuts did not just naturally occur. I reckon there were many makeshift curb cuts that disabled people crafted long before they were recognized. The known US history goes a little something like this: In 1945, Jack H. Fisher petitioned the city of Kalamazoo, Michigan, to carve out sidewalk ramps (read: curb cuts) to allow fellow wheelchair users to cross the street safely. In the late 1960s and early 1970s, a group of wheelchair users, affectionately dubbing themselves "the Rolling Quads," began creating curb cuts all over Berkeley, California. Legend has it that the Rolling Quads took a sledgehammer to existing curbs under the veil of darkness. They didn't wait for permission. Their innovation led the way for the disability rights movement in Berkeley and beyond. When we design with disabled people, all of us benefit.

That's exactly what happened with the sit-to-stand podium. Sure, we designed it primarily with and for wheelchair users, but the podium supported many more people than that. The podium, designed by a small group of people to solve the issue of inaccessibility, became a tool and treasure for more in the community. It became a beacon, not just of access but of possibility.

It's not just the podium. A blind fifteen-year-old developed a six-dot cell system in part to read and write organ music in the 1820s. What was initially used for making music eventually became globally recognized as a communication system for anyone who is blind or low vision, and it is now used in over 130 countries. And all because Louis Braille dared to dream.

In 1808, Carolina Fantoni da Fivizzano, a blind countess, helped produce the typewriter as a way to communicate with her lover. Talk about giving someone the keys to your heart.

Florence B. Seibert, a biochemist who used mobility aids to walk, discovered a way to make injections safer. By eliminating contamination at the injection site, she set a new standard for science and developed a reliable test for tuberculosis that was adopted worldwide. Her interest in the impact of infectious diseases was connected to her own personal experiences of limping after contracting polio.

In the 1950s, before humans were sent to a galaxy far, far away, NASA started recruiting Deaf men from Gallaudet to study the bodymind's response to gravitational environments.[3] Known as the Gallaudet Eleven, these men were never considered astronaut material, but they were instrumental in teaching us how humans react to spaceflight. Zero gravity is no joke. Since congenitally deaf people don't experience motion sickness, NASA wanted to learn from the Gallaudet Eleven how to survive the Vomit Comet. It seems almost too obvious to ask why the Gallaudet Eleven, or other qualified Deaf astronaut hopefuls, weren't considered for any space missions. I fear we already know the answer: *Star Wars: Ableism Strikes Back*.

In 1962, Ralph Braun devised his first motorized wheelchair, before going on to design several more editions. It wasn't just the motorized wheelchair that he developed but wheelchair-accessible vehicles and lifts. The mobility scooter he fashioned is the predecessor of the one I now use. He wasn't just spinning his wheels; he set the wheels in motion for many of us today. I can't imagine my life without Diana, and for her, I and so many other wheelchair users have Braun to thank. Then, in 2010, Stacy Zoern designed an electric vehicle designed for wheelchair users such as herself.

Chieko Asakawa, a blind computer scientist, helped develop digital books using braille, along with text-to-speech translations that are now used for newspapers, articles, and books. Depending

3. Andres D. Almeida, "How 11 Deaf Men Helped Shape NASA's Human Spaceflight Program," NASA, May 4, 2017, https://www.nasa.gov/missions/project-mercury/how-11-deaf-men-helped-shape-nasas-human-spaceflight-program.

on how you are reading this book, you might be using this tech right now. The technology is coming from inside the house. Wanda Díaz-Merced, a blind astronomer, developed sonification, which converts visual data into audible data. Díaz-Merced accounted not just for volume but also for pitch and rhythm in these designs. The access we couldn't write? This is what it sounds like.

In 2011, Farida Bedwei, a software engineer with cerebral palsy, developed a cloud software for microbanking that is now used by 130 finance companies. Her love of programming emerged from using a typewriter and then a computer from a young age as assistive technology. Get that coin, Farida.

Cruise control. Packing tape. The bike. The touch screen. Sensory tools. Rubberized grip on the bottom of mixing bowls. There are so many innovations the disability community has ushered into the world. Long before the world knew these interventions by name, disabled people were crafting and encoding a new creation, often out of the experience of exclusion. We knew the pain of being barred and decided to design a culture of access where we had once been denied. We shared this disability wisdom with one another and found ways to innovate in the midst of it. I want to resist the myth of the singular genius who gets remembered and instead share a mosaic of moments where our community crafted a way where there was no way. I want to honor that there are many more names and narratives that we don't commemorate because they have been erased. Sometimes people will co-opt an idea and act like it was inevitable, but none of these innovations were predestined or predetermined. Each one of them was craftily and cunningly created by and for disabled people, often out of the lived experience of unmet access needs. How many more stories of survival through innovating with duct tape and Popsicle sticks are unknown to us? How many more disabled people are out there crafting new creations in the micro-moments most other people mistake as meaningless?

We aren't done yet. I often find myself wondering what else we could co-create if we were given the chance.

Many disabled people would make great astronauts.[4] Sheri Wells-Jensen argues that crew members would be safer with a blind astronaut who wouldn't be out like a light when it's lights out. Citing how sighted astronauts couldn't find the fire extinguisher when thick smoke clouded their vision during a fire on the *Mir* space station, Wells-Jensen uses her own experiences as a blind person to school us. Blind astronauts wouldn't have had such a sighted plight. Nor would a blind astronaut feel nauseous by the lack of visual horizon that many sighted astronauts suffer from.[5] Houston, we have a solution.

It turns out the final frontier is disabling for all humans. Yet earth doesn't have to be. When we project our ideas about disability onto everything from the way we commune or travel to the moon, we all lose. Imagine what else we could engineer together if we didn't let ableist nonsense deter disabled people from existing as our full selves. The gravity of the situation is that ableism has gone to the moon and back.

I have no interest in becoming an astronaut, but I do care about the assumptions we make about disabled people. All too often we think we know who is disabled and who isn't. Yet the space race can help us trace the ways all bodyminds have access needs that fluctuate based on environment. All too often we assume the worst, when the truth is that disabled people have wisdom and experience to share with the rest of the community. Our experiences and existences, our ways of processing and preparing, our moves and groves, our very beings are gems just the way we are. We shouldn't have to travel to the final frontier for that wisdom to be

4. For examples, check out Ashley Shew, *Against Technoableism: Rethinking Who Needs Improvement* (Norton, 2024).

5. Sheri Wells-Jensen, "The Case for Disabled Astronauts," *Scientific American*, May 30, 2018, https://www.scientificamerican.com/blog/observations/the-case-for-disabled-astronauts.

valued. We are innovators, imagining new ways of being together so everyone can co-flourish.

In our modern moment, innovation is sometimes subsumed by technology. Sure, disabled people have a long history of creating assistive technologies, and will continue to do so.[6] Yet I am not strictly talking about technology when I talk about innovation. These are not the droids you're looking for.

We have developed expertise in finagling access on the fly. Disability wisdom is born of adapting and adjusting in a world that erases and ignores us. Sometimes this is improvised. No curb cut? Take off a shoe and make a makeshift footstool on the go. I can usually stick the landing, but the dismount is a loafer. Batteries low? Find a fellow wheelchair user and get a tow. Left a sensory tool at home? A ring, a zipper, or a rubber band can sometimes do the trick. We know how to transform in the moment, because we've had to. For me, disability has been a generative and expansive reality, helping me forge fresh ways of moving through the world at the drop of a shoe.

Disability has also been a portal to community-building and possibility-making for me. We swap stories of our latest disability hacks. Vibration-only alarms on a phone to reduce sensory overload. A paint stirrer to bridge the small lip in the garage so it's more wheelchair friendly. Bodymaps to reclaim our experiences. Captioning software that knows the difference between "but whole" and "butthole."[7] A rubberized placemat to reduce slippery surfaces. A new way of organizing a fridge that is ADHD friendly.[8]

6. For more on disability dongles, check out Liz Jackson, "Honoring the Friction of Disability," presentation, AIGA Design Conference, April 4–6, 2019, Pasadena, California, available at https://youtu.be/cZhiu-jGbdE.

7. Poet laureate Amanda Gorman's "a country that is bruised but whole" was miscaptioned "a country that is bruised butthole" in her delivery of "The Hill We Climb."

8. For more disability innovations and life hacks, check out Disability at Home at www.disabilityathome.org.

Rubber bands around knobs for easy grip. Reach extenders. Diana holding the bathroom stall closed for me when the lock is broken.

There is an improvisational element to our innovation that is cultivated through necessity. Our expertise is experimental and essential. We share our cultural wisdom with one another in the name of co-flourishing. I am proud to be a part of a community that is deeply creative. My joy in our community isn't toxic positivity. It's not denying what I can't do or proclaiming there aren't challenges in my life because I live in an ableist society that would rather see me dead than divine. It is not #Blessed.

I am proud to be part of the disability community because we are vibrant, innovative, and joyful. I am proud to be a part of a community that accepts me for who I am and tries to meet my access needs. I am proud to be a part of a community that is creative to the core.

Disabled people are the most innovative people I know because we live in a world not made for us. We figure out solutions to problems that nondisabled people are still discovering. Disability is a culture and a community, a way of being that invites us to imagine a new world where all access needs are met without condemnation or critique, where rest is not earned but relished, where we recognize that we move, think, and communicate in diverse ways, and where we know that time is a construct. Disability drives innovation and teaches nondisabled people the inherent wisdom of our disabled bodyminds. We, the disability community, create the future.

PRACTICE

Part of co-creating the world that we want to live in is imagining it and practicing it in our bodyminds. What does a culture of access feel like to you? What does it smell like? What colors are present? What textures? Is it cozy and comforting, like a warm pie? Is it cool, crisp, and clarifying, like a refreshing seltzer on a sweltering day? Are there fuzzy socks and blankets there? Or a hat and sunnies because of the glare?

Spend five minutes imagining a culture of access where everyone can co-flourish. This can be with LEGO blocks, Play-Doh, construction paper, or in a movie in your mind. Think about what it feels like in your bodymind to be part of it, and let's build it together.

3

MY DISABILITY IS INTERDEPENDENT

I have always loved the ocean. I'm from Australia, by way of Southern California, so what can I say? Water is woven into my DNA. The water is where I'd rather be. It soothes and sings; it caresses and comforts; it holds me when it feels like my bodymind is too heavy for this world. Water is my happy place.

But since moving to Washington, DC, I have come to fancy the forest. It all started when I first visited DC before relocating. I was stopped in my tracks one June evening by a light leaping before me. "What is that blinking light? Is that a . . . firefly?" I cautiously quizzed. I had never seen one before, unless you count the Pirates of the Caribbean ride at Disneyland. (I don't.)

There I sat, on the side of the road, yearning for my new, fiery flying friends to burn once more. It's mystical, magical. Once you know, you know.

By the time I moved to the district, summer nights were aglow. I am at peak childhood wonderment when I spot a firefly. "There!" I'd exclaim when one lit up. Another! I'd follow their path as they blinked glitter into the dusky sky. It's nothing short of magical to behold hundreds of them, igniting their incandescent dance to the cue of summer's symphony. Moonbeam ice cream doesn't even come close.

It wasn't just the fireflies. I started to notice something called seasons—a fictional and fanciful fable for an Aussie turned California girlie. I wasn't really acquainted with winter. I knew the concept as a light breeze or a bit of rain that makes you grab a jacket. Read: A jacket in this case is more of a flighty fashion statement than padded protection from the elements. I had traveled to frosty destinations, played in the snow, and knew what it was to feel the kind of bone-chilling cold where your eyelashes and resolve freeze. But there's a difference between stopping by and staying on, and all I had done was visit for a vacation before vacating the wintery premises. Whenever it came to winter, I ghosted. (I've never understood why we say "ghosting" when someone disappears without a trace. Isn't leaving the exact *opposite* of what a ghost does?) Winter was a stamp in my passport, not a home address.

I hadn't lived with the auburn leaves of autumn, the tulips brought by spring, and the singing cicadas serenading us in summer. I hadn't known how sometimes neither salt nor snowplow can contend with winter's grisly grip. Suddenly, I was no longer visiting seasons but *living* them, which, if you think about it, might be more in line with lingering after the after-party like a ghost. Now, I realize that if you are in Michigan, Manitoba, or Mongolia, the concept of DC as a wintery place is likely adorable to you. I get it. I am still learning how to winter. No snowshoes required.

The seasons were brought to life for me by the trees. From cottonwood to redwood, beech to birch, maple to myrtle, trees abound in my neighborhood. The cherry blossoms with their fluffy effervescence, the redbuds whose trunks can't contain their fluorescence, and the ginkgoes with their glorious glow. There are others, but they are not as poplar.

It was the trees that first whispered my worth to me as disabled and divine. I admired their disability: their twisty trunks, contorted branches, and lurching limbs. I knew the trees were here before us and had much to teach us, but I just didn't realize how much. You might say that I couldn't see the forest for the trees.

I started to branch out and spend time admiring the trees every day. "Touch grass," as the youths say. Even savoring their splendor for five minutes to appreciate their lovely leaves, their curved crowns, and their bumpy bark. I liked it most of all when the maple trees kissed in the middle of the road, as if nothing, not sidewalk, street, or stone, could keep them from one another. It seemed like the opposite of a kiss of death, somehow creating life between their caress. The trees generated a canopy of cover and cheer previously unfamiliar to me. I was—and still am—captivated by the trees.

Never more so than when I learned that the trees talk to each other. No, I'm not talking about Groot. Trees are animated throughout Scripture. The trees of the forest clap their hands (Isa. 55:12), argue (Judg. 9:7–15), and shout for joy (1 Chron. 16:33). Trees are lively beings who know how to live in community, often better than us humans do.

Trees aren't just singing and dancing in Scripture. We know that trees share resources, detect danger, and warn one another of looming doom. Like the acacia trees (of the ark of the covenant fame) that emit a distress signal when they sense a giraffe munching on them. A giraffe's chewing starts a signal cycle, where the acacia tree tells all of their friends, "Molly, you in danger, girl!" in the form of ethylene gas. Detecting this SOS, neighboring trees start pumping toxic tannins into their leaves, which, in large enough quantities, can sicken or slaughter giraffes.

It turns out the trees are speaking to each other. Their language? Scent signals. Much like how someone's cologne might offer a whiff of their whimsy or a sniff of their swagger. Right under our noses, trees send signals to one another through scent signs and passing wind.

Acacias are not an anomaly. Pines produce pheromones to entice parasitic wasps when they are under attack from the mighty leaf-eating caterpillar. Tasting the caterpillar's saliva, the pine tree beckons wasps to lay their eggs and feast on the caterpillar, inside out, *Alien* style. In the forest, no one can hear the caterpillar's scream. Oaks pump out bitter bark to dispel insects. It turns out that when a tree falls in the forest and no one is around to hear it, it *does* make a sound. To fellow trees, anyway.

Trees have an interdependent relationship. They are not free-loaders, parasites, or moochers. Deep beneath the ground, tree roots extend more than twice the length of the tree's crown. Fungi become mediators, sharing the latest gossip with neighboring trees. This interconnected communication system transmits signals of drought and danger, nutrients and nourishment, or resources and rejuvenation, from one tree to the next.

Neighboring trees, in turn, change their behavior based on the messages they receive. It's the wood-wide web. Twitter for trees. They are up on the latest from Jenni-fir Lopez, Cate Branch-ett, and Tree-vor Noah. The hum of their gossip carries from root to root. Wise elders nourish impulsive saplings with liquid sugar. Rash youngsters can drink too much, shed too much, and chase after quick fixes and unwise highs (in this case, swift sunlight). I think it's fair to say that doesn't just apply to trees but to human saplings as well. But the sage, aged "mother" trees share their resources so the entire forest can flourish.[1] Wise trees are not in a rush but recognize that slow and steady is sacred. Money doesn't grow on trees, but wisdom does.

Trees even redistribute resources between species. Trees know what humans sometimes forget: that we are part of a community that is reliant on each other. We are better together. Sharing helps maintain biodiversity in the forest and forms an ecosystem that empowers everyone. The trees are not so much interested in survival of the fittest but in survival of the forest. We know that

1. Richard Grant, "Do Trees Talk to Each Other?," *Smithsonian Magazine*, March 2018, https://www.smithsonianmag.com/science-nature/the-whispering-trees-180968084.

God's eternal power and divine nature is displayed throughout the creation (Rom. 1:20). Trees contain—encoded within them and cultivated among them—a divine design for the way the world could be. I wish we could learn from the wisdom of trees how to be interdependent.

"Interdependence" is a slippery term and an even trickier concept. We might praise the idea, but very few of us are taught how to build communities that practice interdependence. Nondisabled people often want to think of disabled folks via a charity model instead, where they have power to bestow or veto whatever money or honey we receive. Typically, this is well meaning, but it comes with a side of shame or snark. Or charity becomes a flimsy friend. If someone supports disabled people out of charity, that behavior will likely terminate when times are tough or when they become too busy. Charity is not a sustainable model of community-building. Try as we might to avoid it, charity still prompts a distance between demographics—an "us" and a "them." The road to interdependence is paved not with charity but with community.

Charity allows for the power dynamic to buttress one person more than another. If you are bankrolling bread or thread for someone, that whips up a power dynamic where it is difficult to foster a genuine, mutual relationship without fear of those resources being revoked. Charity is more about power than personhood. This is likely not our intent, but it happens anyway.

Real interdependence is about community. All people in an interdependent relationship are involved in a love based on giving and receiving as well as having and sharing. And the love they give and have is shared and received. They might not all contribute the same *type* of love: time, talent, or treasure. They might not all contribute the same *amount* of love due to access needs. But they all contribute to creating a community as active participants, not as passive, pitied recipients.

Access intimacy, Mia Mingus explains, is "that elusive, hard to describe feeling when someone else 'gets' your access needs."[2] The beautiful thing about access intimacy is that it understands the fluctuating aspect of access. It happens in mini moments of a friend texting to ask if you still have spoons to meet up that night. Or a coworker naming the access (limitations) of a venue up front so you don't have to carry the burden of additional access labor alone. Or someone suggesting an access check-in. The best part of access intimacy is the chance it offers someone to lift the load of access labor with you. It kindles a connection that is a bridge to building belonging. It means we're not alone and we get to be a part of an interdependent community, much like the wood-wide web.

For me, "community" comes with a lot of baggage. It's a nebulous term that feels at once massive and mundane. It feels like the way many churches use the word "family" to coerce intimacy or to conceal bad behavior. Community feels like a big concept, and it's hard to know if we can ever live up to its demands and expectations. Am I a part of the community if I am excluded? Can I participate in community on some days and not others? Do I count? Some days, I am not even sure which communities really accept or reject me.

One thing I love about access intimacy is how practical it is. We don't need to have done extensive research to bring about access intimacy with one another. We don't need to be experts. We get to show up, with a willingness to learn about one another's access needs, and support one another in meeting them. No saviors or superheroes needed. In short, access intimacy is how we put interdependence into practice.[3] Learning how to meet one another's access needs requires mutuality, flexibility, and consent. It requires understanding one another as image bearers who are a valued part

2. Mia Mingus, "Access Intimacy, Interdependence and Disability Justice," Leaving Evidence, April 17, 2017, https://leavingevidence.wordpress.com/2017/04/12/access-intimacy-interdependence-and-disability-justice.

3. Mingus, "Access Intimacy."

of the community, not charity cases. It's about challenging isolation and independence by cultivating community.

Creating a culture of access where this interdependence thrives welcomes nondisabled people to be a part of our worlds. It invites people into the complexities and chaos of asking for our access needs to be met. It declares, "I'm glad you're here" instead of the typical treatment of demanding our gratitude for the bare minimum (or less). It doesn't require us to shape-shift our access needs for someone else's convenience or calendar. We boldly proclaim that each one of us is worthy of care. Each one of us is a cherished part of the community. Each one of us is loved. Cultivating a culture of access rejects the hierarchies of charity and sows the seeds of a community where we are all interconnected. We put into practice what the trees have long known: We want the entire forest to flourish.

I am always a little weirded out when someone tries to motivate me with odes to independence. "You can do anything you set your mind to! There's no disability except a bad attitude," some pep talks squawk.

Tell that to my legs. Whenever someone tells me there's no limit to what I can do, I wonder if they know about the concept of stairs. Whenever someone tells me they don't think of me as disabled, I wonder why that's the stuff of nightmares. Whenever someone claims I can do anything a nondisabled person can do, I've got to giggle. This is meant to be encouraging, but it is categorically untrue. It only takes about three seconds to realize that.

I understand the impulse to proclaim that I am capable of whatever I set my mind to, but none of us are. There are many things I cannot do because I am human. We make every effort to forget about that part. We tell ourselves the sky's the limit, that we have endless possibilities. We try to perform the myth of our independence. We try to convince ourselves that we are unbreakable.

Look no further than our broken bones to prove this motivational speech a liar.

The truth is, there are many things I cannot do. There are many things *you* cannot do. These might be different things, or they might be the same, but one thing all humans have in common? We are human. And therefore, we are not unstoppable, nor are we gods. We like to insulate our lives from any whisper of dependency or delicacy. We demonize anyone who can't pull themselves up by their bootstraps, erasing the part of the story where we took away their boots. We bank on our bank accounts to inoculate us from our gritty reality. Or we rely on our physical strength or stubbornness to make ourselves believe we *are* pulling ourselves up by our bootstraps, because these boots were made for walkin' and that's just what they'll do. Independence is a core spiritual lie that we often fool ourselves into believing. In my experience, nondisabled people most of all.

But none of us are out here on our own. I have no interest in becoming a #GirlBoss or Miss Independent. I don't just depend on me, and I'm not always 50/50 in relationships.[4] I want to be a part of the community of creation who rely on one another.

The more privileged we are, the easier it is to believe that we are somehow equipped with supernatural powers to be able to do it all, have it all, and be it all. No one seems to want to be human these days. To be human is to admit that you are not God. To be human is to accept that we all have access needs—it's just that some of us are used to admitting it.

Whenever I talk about how we are divine, someone is quick to shut me down or shut me up because we are not God. Amen. I am not God, nor do I want to be. I am human, with all its glorious gunk and junk. We are divine not because we are trying to transcend humanity. We are divine because we are human, made in the image of Creator who taught the trees how to share and the stars how to shine. The trees offer an alternative reality, where

4. Chanequa Walker-Barnes analyzes Destiny's Child's "Independent Women Part 1" on independence as a descriptor and stereotype for Black women in *Too Heavy a Yoke: Black Women and the Burden of Strength* (Wipf & Stock, 2014), 29–34.

interdependence is already an intricate part of the way the world is and the way that we could be. The trees beckon us to belong by sharing our wealth and wisdom with one another.

Interdependence is not all blossoms and beauty. Sometimes interdependence lets us down. Sacrificing and sharing are scary in a system built on scarcity, in a world that extracts. There is a frustration and friction in needing people to meet our access needs and people not coming through for us. I appreciate the wisdom of Naomi Ortiz naming interdependence as "a practice of both loss and of liberation," because both feel true, often in the same moment.[5] It's risky relying on people. Sometimes interdependence falls through not because of malice, or even ignorance, but because life gets in the way. It can be hard to show up for one another when no one is showing up for us. Or we simply don't have the spoons to spend.

Interdependence takes a lot of sacrifice, scheduling, and self-awareness. Setting up who will support the practicalities of life: eating, bathing, and cleaning. Scheduling care. Resolutely carving out pockets of access without the resources to do so. It takes a certain kind of hopeful humility to invite interdependent relationships, knowing they might let us down or leave us out. It is not the stuff of fairy tales.

We are all interdependent, but sometimes it feels like I am *more* interdependent than others. Independence is a type of denial, to be sure, but some of my peers get to fool themselves longer than I do, it seems. There is a reason my shoes don't have laces or why I wear dresses all the time. I often need help with basic needs like putting on my shoes. Some days, that toe-tally socks. Some days, relying on others for basic needs feels heavy and hard.

Yet I have also experienced the way interdependence enriches a connection between us in the way mycelium does, rooting us

5. Naomi Ortiz, *Rituals for Climate Change: A Crip Struggle for Ecojustice* (3Ecologies, 2023), 76.

to one another. There is an intimacy between beloveds when you know how someone likes their food (always more hot sauce!), or where on their backside they want the heat pack (to the left, to the left). There is an intimacy that allows for care to move beyond charity that requires mutual vulnerability. Just as the insistence on independence shuts down the possibility for connection and community, the disability wisdom of cultivating interdependence allows for a depth of intimacy that I have not experienced elsewhere. This intimacy of care and community takes time. Just like the trees sharing their resources, it is a slow go. Interdependent relationships are not built in a day.

The disability wisdom of access intimacy acknowledges that we are fearfully and wonderfully human, and we get the gift of creating communities of care with one another. What if we could be more like the trees, sharing and caring for one another? What if we could remain rooted in our humanity, long enough to admit we all have access needs? What if we could learn from the trees how to become interdependent so we can all thrive? What if we could become vulnerable enough, for long enough, to admit that slow is sacred? Interdependence is evergreen.

One of my favorite stories of access intimacy in Scripture is in Mark 2, when five friends raise the roof off an inaccessible building so one of them can get to Jesus. They dismantle a house that isn't theirs—without permission—because it's not accessible. Take note.

The fab five demonstrate how the inaccessible architecture—not the disabled person—is the problem. In this passage, Scripture is a fan of the social model of disability, which posits that people are not disabled by their bodyminds; instead, the way we nurture community and build environments are what *actually* disables people. A similar construct of disability occurs in many cultures that define disability in relational rather than medical terms or conceptualize disability as diversity. Sandra Yellowhorse has written about how many Diné (Navajo) teachings frame disability within the context of accountable existence to life and land, understanding disability as a communal concept. A Māori understanding of interdependency of space, time, humans, and heritage embraces a variety of bodyminds as part of this broader interconnectedness. Aṉangu culture thinks of disability as difference to celebrate across humanity.[6] Disability has long been considered part of the community in many cultures, in ways the Western world has distorted and destructed. I wonder how much we've disoriented disability in this passage of Scripture as a result.

In church, I learned this passage was about sin; and I think it is, but not in the way I was taught. The passage shows us how to get rid of the sin of architectural exclusion, how to break down the barriers to beloved community, one brick at a time. Whenever someone asks me, "What sin is disabling you?" I want to answer, "Yours!" because I know that the way we have chosen to mold church community—not my bodymind—is what has really barred me from belonging.

There are plenty of ways to get to Jesus: hanging out at wells, fishing, gardening, or taking a dip in the pool. Jesus has also been known to frequent tombs. The fact that these friends dismantled this house calls out the inaccessible structure as the problem. There is no talk of budgets or barriers, no excuses in the form of the intent loopholes, no arguments about who is to blame. Only five friends shredding this inaccessible infrastructure in the name of sacred community.

6. Sandra Yellowhorse, "Indigeneity and Disability: The Teachings of Our Ancestors and Being in Relation Towards Harmonious Outcomes," Disability Visibility Project, June 18, 2023, https://disabilityvisibilityproject.com/2023/06/18/indigeneity-and-disability-the-teachings-of-our-ancestors-and-being-in-relation-towards-harmonious-outcomes; Huhana Hickey and Denise Wilson, "Whānau Hauā: Reframing Disability from an Indigenous Perspective," *Mai Journal* 6, no. 1 (2017): 82–94; and Louis Ariotti, "Social Construction of Anangu Disability," *Australian Journal of Rural Health* 7, no. 4 (1999): 216–22, https://doi.org/10.1046/j.1440-1584.1999.00228.x.

What if we used this passage as a call to action to dismantle inaccessible structures so that everyone can be a part of our communities? If you don't yet consider yourself a part of the disability community, let this image of tearing down inaccessible structures be Scripture's how-to guide for becoming a disability ally. Instead of asking disabled folks to be grateful because we can get in *some* buildings now, or treating us like charity cases, tear down the walls of inaccessibility until no barriers are left behind.

I wonder what it was like, sitting on the roof, ripping it to rubble. I wonder if the fab five felt a thrill or chill while they exposed the ableism of it all. As the five of them worked together to develop access intimacy, I wonder what words and wisdom were passed between them. I wonder who first named the idea aloud, as they shared a fiery glimmer of hope against hope at whether they could actually pull it off. The roof, that is. In my sanctified imagination, I like to picture the disabled man helping hoist his friends up to the roof.[7] I like to visualize the five of them lifting one another as they climbed, supporting each other's weight and access needs as they went. I like to think of the friends as true coconspirators, in it for the long haul. The crew was not there out of charity or convenience. They became like the forest, sharing resources and removing the rubble in one another's paths so that all could flourish.

In this story, the disabled man is not passive or pitied. He demonstrates his own agency and connection to the community. He is under no illusions that he is God. Nor is he treated as an object, outcast from the community of his friends or demeaned as a charity case. Jesus calls him "my child," showing him affection and care (Mark 2:5 NLT).

7. For more on sanctified imagination, check out Katie Cannon, *Black Womanist Ethics* (Wipf & Stock, 1998); and Wilda C. Gafney, *Womanist Midrash: A Reintroduction to the Women of the Torah and the Throne* (Westminster John Knox, 2017), 3.

I love this story because it showcases how a community buttresses a culture of access. Interdependence isn't only for disabled people, of course. It is not solely the responsibility of any disabled person, nor is it rooted in charity. Interdependence is something co-created for the good of the whole. The presence of just one disabled person transforms the community into one where everyone's faith can be strengthened. Everyone gets to experience Jesus in a richer, deeper way because one disabled person was present, encouraging the community to decimate inaccessible structures so that all can get to Jesus. We might say that creating a culture of access with a disabled person offers transformative healing for the entire community, because they are willing to tear down what has been in the spirit of co-flourishing.

I notice a parallel between the fab five dismantling ableist infrastructure and the Rolling Quads, who smashed and dashed their own curb cuts long before the Americans with Disabilities Act passed into law. Unsatisfied with waiting around, both answered the prophetic call by crushing inaccessible structures to create a way where there was no way, to invest in a place where everyone can flourish. Much like the trees, the Rolling Quads are rooted in community care, in the form of curb cuts.

The same can be said for Judy Heumann, Ron Washington, Kitty Cone, and the 150 other activists who occupied the Health, Education, and Welfare Federal Building in San Francisco to implement Section 504 of the Rehabilitation Act of 1973, another precursor to ADA. The 504 sit-ins, as they became known, were supported by Brad Lomax and the Black Panthers, Glide Memorial Church, the Gay Men's Butterfly Brigade, Delancey Street, the Gray Panthers, and the Salvation Army, all of whom provided food, mattresses, and support to disabled protestors. This coalition offered a sustainability that independence could not. People were nourished. Folks used ASL to communicate through the windows when government officials cut off the phone lines. Protestors drew from the cultural wealth of the disability community to outwit government officials by forming their own interdependent forms of communion, communication, and care.

Creating a culture of access is not just in the grand gestures and massive movements; it happens on the small scale and in tiny traces. "Small is all."[8] Slow is sacred. One thing I love about interdependence is that it can happen between two people in a micro-moment. "You are always offering soup," a friend notes one day, surprised by my meal deal after they shared that they were sick. It's true. Yet soup isn't just soup. It's a signal of community care; it practices the beauty of interdependence in a tangible way. Sharing food is disability culture. We show up for one another, one pot of soup or one bag of groceries at a time. Disabled people know what it is to be forgotten, and so we try not to forget others.

Imagine if, instead of trying to change disabled people, we focused our energies on fixing the inaccessible society we have built to exclude people. Imagine if, instead of perpetuating the lie of independence, we followed the trees by practicing interdependence so the entire forest could flourish. Imagine if, instead of bolstering myths of our own independence, we grabbed a sledgehammer, dismantled a roof, brought soup to neighbors, and tore down every inaccessible structure so everyone could thrive. Imagine if we could all get to Jesus.

8. adrienne maree brown, *Emergent Strategy: Shaping Change, Changing Worlds* (Emergent, 2017).

PRACTICE

I have learned so much about my worth from the community of creation. This week, find five minutes to connect with nature in some way. Perhaps you go outside and feel the crisp breeze or warm glow. From a window you might listen to the cardinal sing or the crow caw, or behold the squirrels scurry. Perhaps you let the water hold you. You might graze the texture of a tree's trunk or a pine cone's prickles. Wherever it is, just be. Inhale, exhale, repeat. Let the community of creation declare your connection. Breathe. Be still and know that you are divine.

4

MY DISABILITY IS LONELY

"Sorry you're *huuuuurting*," she consoles, dripping with more compassion for him than a Hallmark card. He offers a meager smile from across the conference table, as if even that is a cluster to muster, given his condition.

His condition? A headache. Not a migraine. Not chronic headaches. Not a throbbing temple that turned out to be something much more traumatic. A simple, nothing-two-ibuprofen-won't-fix headache.

And yet, since this is a nondisabled white man with a headache, everyone's head is spinning. Half a dozen colleagues douse him in sympathy syrup, as though one headache can flatten him like a pancake. Someone even offers to do his share of the work on the team project. Without realizing it, he is workin' it!

Slouched across the table, I try not to slurp my soup in exasperation. Mine is not full of sympathy but of bitter broth. I'm on my fourth week of no solids in between dental surgeries since my teeth keep falling out. Not a dream, a reality of nightmares.

The first time it happened, I blamed the honeycomb. Snap, crackle, pop! Only I wasn't munching Rice Krispies. I was sucking on some honeycomb as I felt the rupture rumble. When I wrenched the wreckage from my jaws, it wasn't just the piece of honeycomb staring back at me but a porcelain spear glistening under the glow of my disbelief.

"Is that . . . my tooth?" I grilled no one in particular.

Glue from the dentist was the only thing holding me together. They cemented the tooth in place, but that was no match for my mighty maw. My mouth was grinding gravel, with only a grave for my molars to show for it. RIP, teeth.

The third time a molar came barreling out of my mouth, my dentist referred me to the endodontist, the big leagues—my biting pain the prerequisite for such a distinguished dentist. I began to think of "DDS" as "dejected dentin society," a joke I was all too ready to tell the dentist when I arrived each time declaring, "I know the drill!"

I've always hated the dentist. Not mine in particular, who seems to have a kind floss-ophy of just trying to send me on my way, toothbrush in tow. It's more the concept of dentists in general. Who wants to stick their hands in everyone else's mouths?

The unforgivable part of the dentist is the awkward attempt at conversation. "How are you?" they probe as your mouth is splayed open, tongue flailing about like you're a snake trying to swallow a moose. "I'm grrrreataaaa," you murmur back, incomprehensibly, wondering how to respond while latex gnashes your gnashers.

So when the dentist explained why we were now seeing so much of each other, all I could manage was a muffled "Whaaaaat?" mixed with the drizzle of my drool, caught only by the trash necklace they force you to fashion.

"It's because your body is in too much pain," I was schooled. "This is your body's way of protecting herself." It felt like he was lying through his teeth. I'm not sure how flicking out my fangs protects me, but okay. My body was taking the whole "tooth for a tooth" thing a little too literally for my taste.

This is how I learned, supine in a dentist's chair one Tuesday before work, that when in enough pain, you can crush and crack your own choppers like a can of soda on your forehead. I wasn't sure whether to be impressed by my sheer strength or hard-pressed by my rejection of myself.

It gave me a lot to chew on. Except for food, of course.

Oatmeal became my menu. Smoothies, my snacks. Solids were off the table for eight weeks while I bore my teeth, hour after hour, and made several treks to the endodontist for them to dig through the nerves in my jaw and re-crown my teeth on their porcelain throne, so that my monarch molars would no longer abdicate their rightful place.

So when my colleague received more sympathy for one headache than I had in the weeks of enduring dental dungeon, it felt a little frustrating to me. I bit my tongue, but it got under my skin. It sent me. It felt like his pain and his pain alone was in italics. I wasn't so bold to expect a little plaque from the dentist, but I yearned for someone to acknowledge my agony. I yearned to be less alone.

Why don't I take something for my pain, one might ask? I'm no stranger to fentanyl or lidocaine. In junior high, I hung out with them more than my friends. It wasn't my peers pressuring me to use drugs as a teenager—it was doctors, shoving them down my throat, writing me off with their prescription pads, wanting my pain to be someone else's problem. Pushing me to pill pop, pressuring me to walk. I'm sure they thought they were justified, because in their minds, walking was so glorified. I learned from that how lonely it is to be in a room full of nondisabled people when you are disabled and in pain.

Whenever people malign that I clutch my pain too closely, I wonder if they realize how they have contributed to this. I am at war. The target: me. I battle myself (not just my molars) about how much to share of my inner life with those around me. I worry that it will be too much, too messy, too excruciating for people to stick around. They'll bail quicker than my molars. So I proceed with caution. I share my pain sparingly, with a spoonful of sugar that is easier for them to swallow. My pain is a nightmare dressed like a daydream. I don't do this out of toxic positivity, humility, or pride. I do this out of survival. I've got a blank space, baby, and I'll hide my pain.

Not all disabled people are in physical or chronic pain. And yet whenever I talk about my pain, it seems to confirm what people already expect: that disabled lives are pitiful and painful, that disabled lives are not worth living, that disabled people are not worth caring about. Pain is a rite of passage for disabled people, or so the thinking goes. No pain, no gain.

Rolling up with a mutilated molar merely confirms people's previous assumptions about disability. I embody everyone's worst nightmare, swaddled in a bedazzled scooter and a smile, stuck together by cement. People expect my life to be full of medical mayhem and painful pasts, so they avoid talking to me all together. They expect that my bark is not worse than my bite. I grit my teeth right up until they fall out.

We adjust our response to how people describe their experience, and I have been in enough pain to know how to manage, mask, and move on. I puree my prickly pain into professionalism so no one notices me wince. That explains why a colleague with a blurt of hurt is shown more sympathy and support than someone dealing with serial stabbing pain that barely registers to anyone else. His pain is making a quick cameo. Mine is the starring role on a syndicated series.

At best, we are met with apathy—at worst, doubt or dismissal—when confronted with our pain. It is like pulling teeth to get anyone to even care. All the while, I realize the one it hurts the most is me. After all, it is my teeth that are off quicker than a bucket of prawns in the midday sun. Being the only publicly disabled person in the room is an isolating experience, full of explanations and excuses. I am lonely. The longer that we are in pain, the less anyone cares about it, and the lonelier we become.

"I feel bad saying it, but I feel uncomfortable around disabled people," one of the pastors confesses, his coffee breath bathing the space between us. I scan the room to find others nodding, lips pursed, with one even praising this pastor for admitting it.

"Grateful we can be honest," one of them reassures him. No one dares to dart their attention in my direction.

We're discussing how to respond to a parishioner who complained that caring about disabled people isn't the gospel, that it makes him frustrated if he can't say ableist slurs around me, that he shouldn't have to "edit" himself at church. He'd called a pastor to whine about me serving Communion because "it's too awkward to have a broken body up there." I had wanted to reply, "This is my body, broken for you," but I thought it would be too on the nose.

It turns out one of our pastors *also* feels uncomfortable with disabled people. Most people are too embarrassed to say that part out loud. I feel it in every stubborn stare, every pity-filled glare, every dismissive pat to my hair, like I am a "good dog," but most pastors don't openly broadcast their discomfort with disability. They camouflage it in Scripture and sanctimony.

I keep waiting for someone to interject, to point out how sinful this is, to act like the disability allies they proclaim to be. I keep waiting for someone to follow Jesus and care about who society deems the least of these. I fear I will always be waiting.

Fast forward to the end of the week, when one of the pastors calls me to check in. He realizes it probably wasn't "nice" for me to know that disabled people make one of our pastors uncomfortable. He means it to be comforting, but it feels cowardly.

I try to explain what it feels like to sit across from someone who casually drops that in a meeting. How it pierces the corner of your soul where your dignity hides—to know that just by existing, you make someone uncomfortable. How lonely it is when others nod along; how gut-wrenching it is to hear Scripture used as a smoke screen for ableism. Words like "ontological" and "image bearer" roll off my tongue, since I know those are the only words that will matter. I dig my fingernails into my palm while I stifle my tears. I am neither pouting nor shouting. I keep my tone level while straining to make an "objective" argument for why I am a full human, as if there is such a thing. It is shattering.

The following week, I go back to the same meeting in the same coffeehouse serving overpriced oat lattes that convince these pastors they are more progressive than they are. I probably shouldn't have, but I still thought I could convince people of my humanity. I still hoped ableism was a function of not understanding. That's that *me* espresso.

And I continued to go back, even when I was told by another pastor that my bodymind was a sign of corruption. "You represent the fall, to remind us that *if* we sin, we could end up like you," this pastor informed me. (*If*, lol.) I went back even when a pastor refused to stop using ableist slurs because those words are in the Bible. Um, okay? If something simply making an appearance in the Bible is the metric for what's moral, have I got news for you. I went back even when I was asked where in the Bible it says we should care about disabled people. I hate to admit it, but I did quote chapter and verse. Again and again and again. I wonder now if there was anything that could have stopped me from going back.

Gracious, they called me. My pastors were quick to praise me as gracious, but what that meant is compliant. So long as they weren't held accountable for their ableism, they tossed around the word "gracious" to make their lack of repentance seem respectable. Everyone loves disabled people until we start asking for our access needs to be met. The day I stopped being their version of gracious is the day I embraced being a full human.

And they reviled me for it. First, it was tone policing. Then came gaslighting masked as Scripture. "Love keeps no record of wrongs" was quoted more than once. Accountability became known by a new name. Holding a grudge, they labeled it. It turns out I was "wounding" my brother in Christ by asking him—in private—to rethink some of his ableist actions. "Brothering" was used to distract from their Othering.

I wish I could say that I knew better than to let it get to me, that I was somehow above it all. But the truth is, it hurts. It hurts to know that my bodymind is a disagreement, a defect, a demonic curse to many who call themselves my siblings. It hurts to realize that no amount of proximity or personality can convince people that my mere existence isn't a mistake. It hurts to know that there is nothing I can ever do or say to endow myself with humanity in their eyes.

It hurts to be half human.[1]

This is a common routine that has played on repeat throughout my life. Step 1: Disabled people start sharing our access needs and the ways we're currently excluded. Step 2: Some nondisabled people get defensive and blame us as the problem. Now let me see you, one, two, step. Here we go!

Until the revolutionary becomes routine, the change agent is often blamed. I am cast as the mischief maker, the chaos culprit, the rabble rouser. I've been told that I shouldn't get "swept up" in advocating for access, as if justice is a broom. Several churches warn me not to make "such a big deal" about access, because it makes others feel bad when I bring it up. Whether it's in the workplace or a church space, I carry the weight of this inaccessibility and ignorance on my shoulders knowing that—when it comes to

1. Amy Kenny, "It Hurts to Be Half Human," *Preach*, May 9, 2022, https://www.preachweb.org/blog/half-human.

access—no matter what I do, no matter how much I smile, or how I beguile, I'm the bad guy. Duh.

I have chosen to be kind over curt. I have chosen to be joyful over jaded. I have chosen to invite people in instead of canceling people out. And I have been condemned as the problem anyway.

My biggest sin of all has been disrupting the unity, they say. I am making the church look bad for pointing out its flaws. News flash: Unity was never there in the first place. Uniformity and unity are not the same thing. I never meant to start a war. I just wanted the church to let me in. All I wanted was to take a wrecking ball to the walls of ableism, but instead, it wrecked me.

I am not criticizing one corrupt leader but the collective culture that disciples this ableism to become pervasive in our churches. The uncomfortable truth is that once you are on a journey of justice, many people will revile you for it. People will tell you to stop in the name of protecting you or even loving you. People will stop talking to you. Others will directly dismiss anything you say as "too activist," "too touchy," or "giving the devil a foothold." And many of those people will be the same ones who speak loudly about Jesus or justice.

I know because some churchgoers did it to me. Speaking up for disabled people has lost me community and opportunities; it has caused tension and trauma; it has devastated me when I thought I had no more tears left to cry. It has cost me more than I thought I was willing to give. I haven't always known when to roll away or how much to raise in the moment. I am lonely, languishing for the church to care. I am lonely, despite knowing so many have endured this shut up and kiss-off from the church.

I want to believe that disabled people are excluded not from malice but from neglect. But most days, the reason doesn't really matter to me all that much, because I am excluded all the same. It is hard to be a part of a community when you have been so neglected that even reminding people of your existence does not cultivate change. I am lonely, even in a group of so-called allies. I am all by myself, and I don't want to be all by myself anymore.

People are quick to remind me that Jesus was lonely, borne of betrayal from people meant to be buddies. That he endured the ultimate kiss-off. I know that there can be something holy even in the hurt, but that does little to make me feel less alone. I feel betrayed, all the while being accused of betraying the very church I am investing in changing. I am no Jesus, Judas, or Jedi. I am just a girl, sitting in front of the church, asking them to love us.

"They shouldn't have invited you!" she sighs.

The words spiral between us like a roller coaster I did not ask to be on. *She mustn't have said that,* I try to reassure myself, determined not to descend into despair. I'm recounting an event I couldn't attend because it was not accessible. Two stairs were the only barrier barring me from belonging. After I shared with my friend how dehumanizing it was to get to the event and be turned away, she tries to mollify me by suggesting that I shouldn't have been invited in the first place.

Somehow, that's not the solution I was hoping for. Excluding me ahead of time doesn't excuse excluding me on the day. After I pointed out that claiming something is inaccessible doesn't give someone a get-out-of-jail-free card, she retreats. We are at a stalemate.

I am alone again, naturally.

I ask my church if the building we're moving to has an accessible entrance so I can participate. I'm told to stop asking about access, because it's "just" me who is disabled, not the community. The word "just" is said with all the emphasis of a scowl.

I am alone again, naturally.

I break away from the crowd so I can make it to the accessible entrance at the back of the building. The group saunters in the front, up the stairs to the service. I hustle past the entrance, wind around the wingspan of the expanse, and hoof it to a different building just to slip in the door and sit by myself, the accessible seats separated from everyone else. It's only ten extra minutes, but the distance between me and the rest of the community is light-years. I want to be out of my inaccessible era. I must travel four times as far to get half as much.

I am alone again, naturally.

I ask the pastor to stop describing disability as uniquely sinful. He tells me that I need to be patient because not everyone will be okay with that. When I ask how long I should be patient, he sneers like I'm a lost mutt in need of a home. Woof.

I am alone again, naturally.

I sit in yet another Wednesday night gathering where a disability slur is used and no one says anything. When I bring it up, I'm told I'm being divisive. Dividing what, exactly?

I am alone again, naturally.

I listen in agony as a friend is reprimanded for addressing ableism because of the tone of her voice. It's like that annoying feeling when you know there's a fly in the room but can't seem to spot it. Only its unnerving zzz echoes around the room. Addressing ableism is almost always treated as more of a problem than the ableism itself. Ableist nonsense buzzing everywhere.

I am alone again, naturally.

I am lonely. I don't mean that I need more friends. As an introvert, I genuinely prefer the company of a book over a person. (No offense, beloveds.) I'd rather spend my time thinking about how "you cooked" (good) and "you're cooked" (bad) came to be than cook a meal with a bunch of cooks.

I adore my companions and confidants, and I am at peace when it's me, a party of one. When I say I am lonely, I don't mean I want more followers or friends. I mean that I feel alone in creating a culture of access in many communities that I call my own. I am lonely because I am usually the only one to speak up or take up access labor.

Disability is so often last, least, or left out. Even among people who are interested in creating a more just world, disability is just so often neglected. I get it. Disabled people have been segregated from society, and it's difficult for people to remember someone they didn't know they forgot. But some days, when I have enough courage to let myself cook, I wish I wasn't so lonely.

Inaccessibility is an accepted form of bias. Many of us have decided that it's acceptable to exclude disabled people, so it no longer shocks or rocks people. It's giving all the care of the automated operator repeating, "Your call is very important to us" for the fifth time while on hold with your insurance company. After a while, it starts to feel like your call *isn't* that important. Patience is called for from disabled people when we have very little left to give. I wish the weight wasn't so heavy. I wish the wait wasn't so long. Why do I need to be patient with their prejudice?

It is draining to absorb everyone's embarrassment at creating inaccessible spaces, day after day, party pooper after access blooper. Ableist nonsense prevails. What's more, most people assume an individualized model of accessibility, which presumes that I and I alone am "the problem." It makes *me* the issue instead of what it really is: a potent potion of inaccessibility in the built environment and demeaning attitudes. It conveniently leaves out the part where we choose to exclude members of our community physically, digitally, or attitudinally. Inaccessibility produces isolation.

We choose to build spaces inaccessibly. We choose who gets to be a part of the community. We choose who is in and who is out. Even without meaning to, we decide who belongs. Very few people seem to care or know about disability, and some people like it better that way.

All of this is by design, for the simple fact that stairs are not naturally occurring. Humans put them there. There are no stairs on the bike path, on the train tracks, or in the bus lane. Yet when it comes to a building, we toss in some stairs for good measure. Why, tho? Never mind that bikes, buses, trains, and cars all use wheels to get around. It's only wheelchair users that we've deemed unsound. That makes about as much sense as paying for an escape room when you can go to IKEA for free.

The good news is that, just as we built this world the way it is, we can *re*build it in a different way. Nothing needs to be "just the way things are." We do not have to suffer communities where people are lonely for being who they are. We do not have to endure spaces that erase the beautiful diversity of the community of creation. We do not have to be alone again, naturally.

I bet the prophets were lonely. We don't have to look far to figure out why. Samuel pulled a *Casper* just to bad-mouth Saul. Talk about an unfriendly ghost. Elisha was bald and summoned bears to maul any mockers. Seems a bit emotional. When his precious gourd plant withered, Jonah hit the roof. Oh my gourd, just chill, mate. Isaiah walked around naked. Jeremiah hid his underwear in the river. Ezekiel gave himself a haircut with a sword before setting some of his hair on fire. That's a bit dire. He also baked his barley cakes over human dung. Mmmm . . . it must have been fragrant. (Did I say fragrant? I meant flatulent.)

The prophets, as a group, seem more like party-poopers than crowd-pleasers. They aren't exactly at the top of the invite list. It's not profitable to be a prophet either. No wonder prophets aren't accepted in their hometown. Beneath the emotional roller coasters and community roasters, I bet they were lonely.

So it's not particularly flattering when your church calls you a prophet. My church community did, until I asked them to learn about disability theology and then was cast aside like yesterday's dung.

I had let myself hope that my church at the time was different—that when the time came, we would practice what we preached. Instead, I found myself wounded and weary, wishing for the label of "prophet" to not have turned out to be so painful. Perhaps that's why I find myself drawn to the prophets. I am mesmerized by these wild and wacky details of their lives. Why include them? Why preserve all the gnarly goss? Why tell us what loners they were?

I wonder if it makes them all seem more like wonderful weirdos instead of winners. I wonder if this allows them to resonate with so many of us who are cast aside as weird but are really just limited edition. How many of them were disabled but labeled as "weird" in the pages and on the stages of history? I wonder if this is just another reminder that God cares for whomever society deems to be the lost, the last, the least, and the left out. I wonder if these unsavory signs help us understand something about how even our loneliness can be divine.

Walter Brueggemann describes the prophet as one who is called "to nurture, nourish and evoke a consciousness and perception alternative to the consciousness and perception of the dominant culture around us."[2] As Andre Henry says, "It doesn't have to be this way."[3] Prophets aren't merely applying timeless standards to The Discourse™ but offering an interpretation of a divine

2. Walter Brueggemann, *The Prophetic Imagination*, 2nd ed. (Fortress, 2001), 3.

3. Andre Henry, "It Doesn't Have to Be This Way," released October 10, 2017, https://andrehenrymusic.bandcamp.com/track/it-doesnt-have-to-be-this-way.

understanding of our particular moment. "Prophecy, then, may be described as exegesis of existence from a divine perspective."[4]

Or, to put it plainly, the prophet's role is to alert people that we are in the Upside Down in *Stranger Things*. Sure, it might look like Hawkins High. It might even seem like Scoops Ahoy. But this is not the real deal. Taste and see that the ableism is not good. The prophet's role is to criticize the way things are and energize the community into imagining a different way the world could be. Prophets aren't naysayers for negativity's sake. They point to a different way, full of compassion and community. Perhaps their loneliness can help us understand that instead of the gluttony of greed, we can focus on generosity. Instead of the idolatry of independence, we can foster interdependence. Instead of discarding disabled people, we can cultivate collective access for all of us. Instead of becoming jaded, we can pursue justice.

We are not here to dictate the divine or to dole out dignity. We are not here to determine who is in and who is out, who is celebrated and who is shamed, who is encouraged and who is tamed. As the prophet Rachel Held Evans reminds us, "What makes the gospel offensive isn't who it keeps out, but who it lets in."[5] And whether we like it or not, whether we realize it or not, disabled people are already in.

Disability is an experience that defies the hierarchies that humanity has handed to us. It's often hard for people to come to terms with the divinity of disability, because it makes us reckon with our sense of self. It makes us realize that many of us have been in the Upside Down all along.

Disability activist and MacArthur "Genius Grant" fellow Alice Wong calls disabled people oracles, because we are often the first

4. Abraham J. Heschel, *The Prophets* (Perennial, 2001), xii.

5. Rachel Held Evans, *Inspired: Slaying Giants, Walking on Water, and Loving the Bible Again* (Nelson, 2018), 186.

to alert everyone to incoming doom.[6] But we are not just mythical figures with potent potions and tarot cards foretelling what looms. We are here, now, asking the church to love us. We are so often alone in pleading for the access so many of us are needing. Disabled people are prophetic because we nourish new worlds that are built for our bodyminds, communities where we can co-flourish. Come and join us in making such a world a reality.

The prophets are not brilliant wizards condescending to the people from on high. They are down in the muck. Their bodyminds are a part of their prophetic witness, and ours are too. I bet they wondered how they would go on. I bet they were drained from being outcasts. I bet they were tired. I bet they were lonely, but disabled people don't have to be.

On days when I feel loneliest, I open my phone. (Not to Twitter. Never to Twitter.) I read a note full of memorable moments from trusted truthtellers. There's one sentence from a friend, thanking me for showing up for her. There's another from a disabled churchgoer who used my book as a catalyst to advocate for infrastructural changes at their church. There's a photo of a jacaranda's purple snow powdering the pavement, basking in the sunlight. These are small but mighty reminders that I am not alone, even though it often feels like it. The whole community of creation declares our divinity.

If you are disabled, you might feel lonely too. Maybe one way we remind ourselves that we are not alone is by practicing the way we show up for each other. We show up every time we call someone in or call someone up to check on them. We show up with soup in hand or push pops in tow. We show up every time we cheer one another on. We show up every time we live our magnificent disabled lives to the fullest. We show up when we name our pain of being lonely.

We are not alone, even if we are lonely.

6. Alice Wong, "Message from the Future: Disabled Oracle Society," Disability Visibility Project, August 14, 2020, https://disabilityvisibilityproject.com/2020/08/14/message-from-the-future-disabled-oracle-society.

PRACTICE

We are not alone, even when we feel lonely. When I am lonely, I try to remind myself that we are interconnected. Inspired by Stacey Park Milbern and Alice Wong's work on crip ancestors and lineage, I create a constellation map of beloveds. These beloveds can be people who are in my past or present communities, or elders and ancestors who I am connected to in spirit. There are no rules about who you can include. If you feel connected, they are a part of your constellation. Try writing the names of people who make you feel less lonely on the constellation map below.

You are connected to a constellation of communities, even when you are lonely. You are not alone.

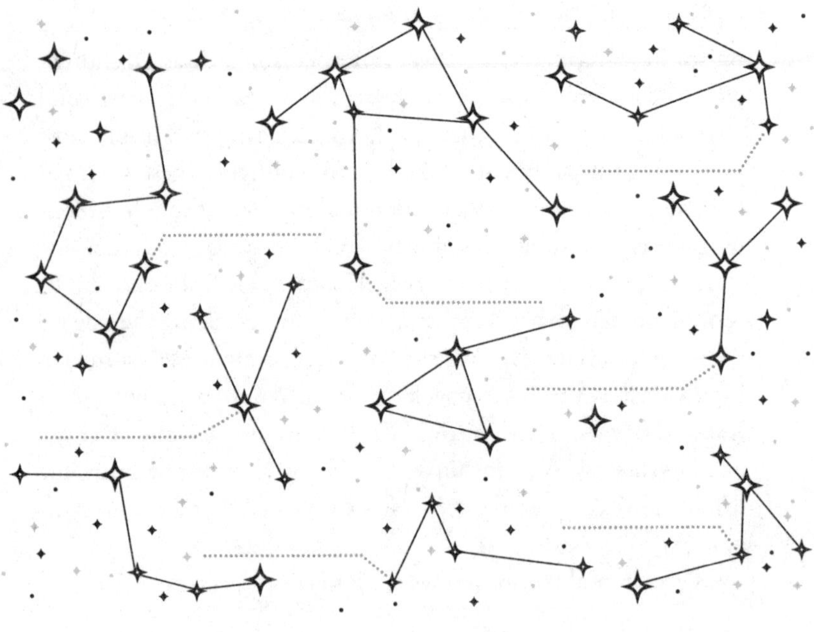

5

MY DISABILITY IS PROPHETIC

We were brushing our teeth when it happened. Our minds were preoccupied with the midweek minutiae of making it out the door to my 8 a.m. class and his 7:30 a.m. meeting. Neither of us made it on time.

"Do you think there's any chance it could fall on us while we sleep?" I asked my spouse, Andrew, the night before while we were untucking the sheets. It seemed like the ceiling just got some bad news; it was drooping. My drowsy eyelids zoomed in on the sag slacking around the fan, but I reassured myself that it was just my weary perspective from the bed below.

"Ceilings *shouldn't* fall," Andrew did his best to reassure both of us. I now realize "shouldn't" is doing a lot of work in that sentence. Too much heavy lifting.

Our air conditioner had just been replaced. During another grueling summer with an AC older than we are, we had finally taken the plunge. Wednesday had come with cool air, brought to us by a crane installing the unit on top of our unit, right above our bedroom.

It's hard to sleep with a saggy ceiling above your bed, but I had coached myself that nothing was gained by my awning fawning and tried to ignore my sinking ceiling feeling. The next morning, while brushing our teeth, the ceiling collapsed right between us. We were on either side of the bed, doing the sunrise shuffle. It turned out that the AC company was full of hot air.

A four-foot-by-five-foot chunk of our roof plummeted to rest on the bed, with mounds of mushy insulation in its wake. A chunky ceiling slushy was not the breakfast I had in mind. Somehow, the fan was still steadfastly dangling overhead, taunting us with each spin. Do I need to spell it out? I was not a fan.

There was nothing Andrew or I could do but laugh. We gazed across the debris at one another, quickly assessing that neither of us was hurt, before bursting into a belly laugh that only comes by way of soggy ceiling slump.

The AC company hadn't installed the air conditioner correctly, glugging gallons of water onto unsuspecting drywall. It was an honest mistake. Our housed friends rapidly recommended that we sue the AC company, a suggestion that came on like indigestion. Suing and slamming were more of a priority than supporting. But we weren't interested in suing, just pursuing a repair.

The thing about being in community with disabled folks, many of whom are unhoused, is that it shifts your perspective. Many of our unhoused neighbors offered material support—food, clothes, a personal fan—anything we might need while our roof was restored. Our housed friends were concerned with chastising; our unhoused friends concentrated on community. Our housed friends were focused on retribution; our unhoused friends wanted restoration. Our housed friends wanted us to be independent. Our unhoused friends wanted to make sure we were cared for. The gap was massive, much like the hole in our ceiling.

Less than two months later, a pipe burst. Our collapsed ceiling had been replaced, only for a bigger collapse that couldn't be fixed with some drywall and a bucket of eggshell. Gray water creeped and seeped through the bathroom before taking out the living room. Think Beyoncé opening the floodgates in *Lemonade.* Water gushed from floor to door. That night, we moved out with a couple of T-shirts in a duffle, expecting to return in a few days. That's what the contractor told us, anyway. They'd fix the damaged pipe, nix the dirty floor, and with two clicks of our ruby slippers, there'd be no place like home, forevermore.

It was more than four weeks until we moved back in. Water is quick and slick. It knows no barrier, no border, no bounds. Its contamination compounds. We spent the holidays in a local extended-stay place, where breakfast was included in the nightly rate (score!), while our condo was stripped to the studs and sterilized. Our Thanksgiving was underwater. Our place quit us, cold turkey.

One Wednesday night, while I stopped by to collect fresh clothes, our neighbor paused her "Christ alone" track just long enough to come over and yell at me about the racket generated by the repairs. "You need to pay for a hotel for me at the beach until this is done," she demanded.

I apologized for the inconvenience. I had a nasty bout of viral laryngitis at the time, so I mainly listened. I listened when she blamed me for the interruption to her TV schedule. I listened when she claimed that our leak—confined to our condo—caused her weeping, so much weeping, it was sweeping emotional distress. I listened when she demanded we rush the remediation, as if we had the power to do anything but wait. And I listened when she attempted to commit insurance fraud by trying to force us to foot the bill for her elective bathroom renovations. The moment she shut her door, "This gift of love and righteousness" blared through the walls yet again.

The following Sunday afternoon, we met up with our friends at the laundromat. About thirty people who are unhoused or housing insecure make up our crew. Most of them are disabled. Many of them have been discarded and become homeless *because* they are disabled (or what we sometimes label it in polite company: medical bankruptcy). We used to meet at the local park for a chili potluck, but we got kicked out after too many people called the cops on us for befriending folks who are unhoused. The city even commissioned a local pastor to explain why loving our neighbors was dangerous, because people were "taking advantage." Who wouldn't want to take advantage of "this gift of love and righteousness"? Concerned about the growing backlash to our unhoused neighbors, we pivoted to the laundromat across the street.

Boxes of pizza in one hand and a jar of quarters in another, we hang out with our friends experiencing homelessness; folding clothes, swapping stories, and singing to the classics that Mr. Lee blares a little too loudly. The laundromat has become the backdrop to many a spontaneous rendition of "Sugar Pie, Honey Bunch," with more mirth than melody.

There's no formal mission or ministry at the laundromat. It is not a charity or a crusade. It's just a couple of friends, with pie and a jug of Tide, showing up to build community with our neighbors. We love in the form of clean clothes, full bellies, and interdependent community care. Newbies are often expecting a lecture, or at least a liturgy, when they first come to the laundromat. Instead, we hand over a slice and help each other fluff and fold.

Over a piece of pepperoni, I chatted with Matt, one of our regulars. Matt would make a great Santa Claus. Between his sparkling eyes, his hearty laugh, and his jolly demeanor, he was a shoe-in for Kris Kringle. That is, if he could wear shoes. Matt was always rocking sandals since his ankles, swollen by medical neglect, couldn't squeeze into the likes of shoes anymore, which he'd tell you behind a soulful chuckle. When we'd ask him if he needed any support that week, he'd tell us a random, unrelated fact. Sometimes, it was about his white German shepherd, Alexander. Other times, it was a new book rec he'd learned from someone's uncle on Facebook. Or the snot-based home remedy that he swore by, that we all teased him about. You may think it's funny, but it's snot.

"You back at home yet?" Matt asked, with a familiar grin. When I told him we weren't, but we were all good, he asked if we needed anything. He offered his gray blanket and reassured us that he and Alexander would look out for us if we needed his help.

There we were in our local laundromat, with washing machines whirling all around us, being taken to church. "Christ Alone" wasn't playing, but he was present. Our friends who are unhoused cared more about supporting us than searching for someone to blame.

Whenever I think about the Great Banquet (Luke 14:15–24), I think about our community at the laundromat. In this parable, Jesus tells us the kingdom of God is a feast, full of disabled and poor people, and there is enough for everyone. No lawsuits or neighbor disputes, no being chewed out by rude neighbors, just delicious food where everyone gets enough to eat. To quote the youths, we ate.

I have experienced more community with my disabled, unhoused friends than I have in any other church I have been a part of in my life. People bicker and belittle, to be sure. There have been heated fists and cold shoulders. Accusations and arguments about parking spots are aplenty. See also: "You're not playing dominos with *him*, are you? I thought you were *my* friend!"

But underneath the parking spot spats and the domino drama is a camaraderie cultivated only in genuine community. People regularly share what little they have so no one goes without. At the park and the laundromat, folks have everything in common, often out of necessity, messily.

I have witnessed friends dish out their last bowl of chili, wash someone else's stuff, or fetch a toothbrush or a tampon when a friend can't make it. I have taken advantage of their kindness. I have witnessed our community's generosity toward one another and toward me countless times: the Christmas card that each of them signed ("Girl, you *riding* that scooter!"), the turquoise mug they gifted me because it's my favorite color, the offer of food during peak pandemic when Andrew's event-based salary was reduced by 40 percent, and the friendship formed, one bowl of chili or slice of pie at a time.

Our friends take their copper mite and share it. It's not just their two cents; they watch each other's tents. They save one another a space to park and spot each other's stuff in the dark. They shuttle one another around the city. Their love isn't just an abstract notion or a Bible verse, it's nitty-gritty. Sometimes it ain't pretty. But they look out for each other when there are surly neighbors and nightly sweeps. It is no picnic—except for when it's a literal picnic at the park—but interdependence runs deep in the community that is cultivated at the park turned laundromat. No doubt, they have our backs. And we have theirs.

I feel safer with my unhoused, disabled friends at the park than I do with most housed churchy folks, because I have witnessed how much good fruit their faith bears. We don't have to pretend to be nondisabled at the park or mask our own access needs. We don't have to put on a poker face or save face to fit in. We get to show up, fully as ourselves, and belong. There is no bickering over beliefs or splintering over details of doctrine. We might not use words like "theology" and "mutual aid," but we practice it. All of us can just be. The hard truth is that most of the time, the park and the laundromat is more church than church—as well as more community than my neighbors were during the round-robin of repairs.

We shared a street, but little else. Where we lived at the time—a condo community within strolling distance to Froyo and PetSmart—was hollow compared to the hallowed vibrancy of community at the park. Sure, we had a roof over our heads (that sometimes collapsed) and a place to shower (that sometimes burst), but we didn't have the radical goodness between us, the genuine love between neighbors that means you love one another as yourself. The type of care that shares what you have with one another, even down to your last blanket, because you have everything in common. I think I read about that community practice somewhere (Acts 2:44–45).

At the park, people are known, really known, for who we are—attitude, anger, addiction, access needs, and all. Our neighborhood was full of manicured lawns and manicured hands waving hello to nameless neighbors as they walked their dogs, but there was no real community in the community. Each neighbor went about their lives as if independent from the whole. Sometimes we knew one another's government names, but we didn't know one another's stories. We didn't really know each another, not enough to give each other a nickname. Not enough to really love one another.

Some of us might have been loved by a church congregation at some point in our lives, until . . .

we asked for an access need to be met
we came out
we asked a question we're not "supposed" to ask
we got divorced
we went to a protest
we became homeless
we voted for the *other* party
we stimmed
we *didn't* have kids
we dared to be different

If our churches extend community care only to people who are exactly like us, what good are we (Luke 6:32–36)?

On the whole, the white American church has so often confused selfishness with self-reliance, hoarding with helping, and #Blessed with wealth-obsessed. Instead of storing up treasures in heaven, we hoard them in our houses. Instead of sharing, we're stockpiling. Instead of cultivating a practice of care, we accumulate more and more and more until we're so full of our own self-determination that we are no longer hungry for justice. Where your treasure is, your heart will be also, and for many in the white American church, our treasure is more easily located in a tax shelter than a homeless shelter.

If we have a church but don't have love, we are bankrupt, nothing but clanging gongs of greed and cymbals of self-reliance. We can change the way things have been and tend to a community of care where all of our access needs are met, where all of us can co-flourish. Let us repel the moths of materialism and the rust of oppression from rotting our communities away. Church, we are listening to the wrong profits/prophets.

So many of us have found ourselves cast out of a church that was never made with us or for us, a "church" that values white supremacy, queerphobia, misogyny, ableism, and classism more than the image bearers in our beloved community. Many of us have changed teams but still practice the same routines of factions and retractions. We seem to think we're called to cancel. Many of us are more active in outrage culture than cultivating support for outcasts. Many of us still think in "us" versus "them" when we are all image bearers. And yet as Sarah Bessey reminds us, "I want to be outside with the misfits, with the rebels, the dreamers, second-chance givers, the radical grace lavishers, the ones with arms wide open, the courageously vulnerable, and among even—or maybe especially—the ones rejected."[1] Friends, there is no place I'd rather be.

This is a prophetic way of living, brought to you by whomever society deems the least of these. My disabled, unhoused friends gave out of their poverty, much like the widow giving her last coin. Their prophetic witness made what is true feel more real. It brought priorities into focus. It didn't matter where we were living; what mattered is that we had somewhere cool and dry to lay our head at night without fear for our safety (or a ceiling somersault). What

1. Sarah Bessey, *Jesus Feminist: An Invitation to Revisit the Bible's View of Women* (Howard, 2013), 3.

mattered is that we were cared for. Our community was not there to teach us a lesson or make us grateful; they were there to be a community, with all of its complicated and confounding realities.

Our housed church friends didn't know how to meet and support our access needs outside of threatening retaliations or lawsuits. Maybe this is because our unhoused friends are practiced at supporting one another's access needs and realize the value of interdependence. Maybe this is because disabled people know what it feels like when our own access needs are not met. Whatever the reason, disabled, unhoused people knew how to be a part of a community not of hierarchy but of humanity. Our friends knew that we are all inherently valuable, regardless of how we choose to organize society.

At the laundromat, we cultivate a culture of access. People show up and support one another's fluctuating needs. Everyone participates in wildly different ways based on their own needs. It is messy and chaotic, and it is beloved. It is a thin place where we can meet the divine.

As much as I have been loved and cared for in this community, I wish life was not this way. The American church has the power to end homelessness, yet we choose not to.[2] Disability is so often the cause and consequence of homelessness. I do not want to glorify or gloss over our call to action when it comes to caring for our neighbors whom society has cast the least, the last, and the left out. I think Jesus would have a lot to say about that. I also don't want to reduce the complexities of our disabled lives to moralizing ideas of learning lessons, as though we were all living Aesop's fables. Life is much more complicated than that. But I do think the church can learn from the prophetic witness of our communities. I know I have.

The disability community is prophetic because we often reveal what is true about humanity. At the park, people are embraced not

2. For more on what the church can do to end homelessness, check out Kevin Nye's book, *Grace Can Lead Us Home: A Christian Call to End Homelessness* (Herald, 2022).

because of who we pretend to be or even for what we can offer one another, but because we are a cherished part of the community. That's it. That's the message. Imagine if the church could be more like the park and less like the angry neighbor. The church could be full of characters who have nothing in common on paper but who choose to cultivate community in practice. Maybe then we could love one another as ourselves. Maybe then we could actually *be* church instead of just going to church.

We can't go back, but we can go beyond. When we start to believe we are all worthy of life and life abundantly, we change the way we interact with the world. We know that we don't have to hoard, but can help one another. We know that our liberation and joy are connected to one another's, and even to members of our communities who we pretend are not like us. When we really believe this, we no longer think of a culture of access as the stuff of fantasy but know that it can be reality. We know that a world where our access needs are met and where we are worthy of care is not fictional, it is factual.

I hope against hope that we find ourselves in such communities. Until we do, let us pick up some pizza, grab a handful of quarters, and head to the local laundromat. Maybe there, we will find Christ—not alone but in community with outcasts whom society has deemed the least of these. Maybe there, we can learn from the prophetic witness of unhoused, disabled people what it means to enrich a community where all can co-flourish.

We hold these truths to be self-evident, that all humans are created with access needs, and that we are endowed by our Creator to certain unalienable rights, that among these are life, liberty, and the pursuit of access. This is my Declaration of Interdependence.[3]

3. For more on a declaration of interdependence, check out Lachi, *I Identify as Blind: A Brazen Celebration of Disability Culture, Identity, and Power* (Tiny Reparations, 2026), 265.

We all have access needs. An access need is anything someone needs to be able to fully participate in a community. Access needs can be related to the built environment in both physical and digital landscapes, language, lighting, communication, chemicals, social media, pace, processing, temperature, food, rest, and more. All of these are part of the same song, just different verses.

Too often when we talk about access, people just want to sing, "Let's get physical" but not, "Digital, digital get down" or, "I've got a new attitude." Not all access needs are *treated* equal. Some are considered bona fide, while others are labeled fake. Some access needs are branded extra or excess. We all need somewhere to pee. Yet bathrooms are only provided for some of us. We all need food that nourishes. Yet some dietary access needs are berated as burdens or bonuses. People generally have a different disposition to service animals than stimming. Service animals are considered cute and cuddly. Cue the chorus of "Aww!" Who's a good boy? Yes, you are!

Stimming to process internal body signs is usually cast as weird at best or dangerous at worst. We've come around to accepting *some* stim tools (read: fidget spinners), but generally, we're dismissive of this access need. We're so convinced that someone is acting contrary or scary, particularly if that someone is an autistic Black person.[4] But push pops are not to be pushed aside. Chewies are not to be chewed out. Tangle toys are not worth getting twisted over. All of these are needed tools that meet access needs.

Many of us stim without realizing it. We call it clicking a pen, licking a lollipop, tapping our feet, playing with rings, or snapping our bracelets. Regardless of whether we identify as neurodivergent, we can learn from the wisdom of using sensory tools to process our internal body signs. In this way, the disability community offers a prophetic witness for creating a community with less masking

4. Black bodyminds are more likely to be interpreted this way. For more, check out Sami Schalk, *Black Disability Politics* (Duke University Press, 2022).

and blasting and more of a culture of access everlasting. Our access expertise and disability wisdom can benefit everyone. We invite the ways that disability disrupts our constrained notions of what community can be.

So often, disabled people are met with disability doubters and additional access labor just to get in the door or pace the floor. Our bodyminds absorb the additional access labor of navigating a world not built for us. We are asked intrusive questions about our bodyminds, pressured to proclaim personal details about our access needs or medical records. We are often made to feel obligated to accept unwanted touch without consent. We are treated as burdensome for having access needs at all.

Disabled people are regularly expected to broadcast the deepest crevasses of our experiences, without many people realizing this is humiliating.[5] Whenever I've asked people to stop forcing us to expose the deep-seated details of our lives, they reply that they are *trying*. Do or do not, there is no try.

Too often when we talk about access, people are quick to make excuses of what costs or what counts, as if you have to be disabled "enough" to have access needs. People are quick to tell me that historical buildings can't become accessible because they were built *before* the Americans with Disabilities Act. So they're telling me that we can't expect an old building to be accessible because it was constructed *before* we considered disabled people a part of the community. Did I get that right?

Somehow, I've never heard the same argument for indoor plumbing, air conditioning, or Wi-Fi. Whenever I point out that historical buildings *could* become more accessible, that's where people draw the accessibility line. It is clear that we are used to valuing disabled people less than some old columns and cobblestones.

5. For more on this, check out Mia Mingus, "Forced Intimacy: An Ableist Norm," Leaving Evidence, August 6, 2017, https://leavingevidence.wordpress.com/2017/08/06/forced-intimacy-an-ableist-norm.

We disable people by the way we set up the environment, then cobble anyone who dares to ask for access. It's exhausting. Perhaps some of what makes community at the park and the laundromat is that time is usually not wasted on bickering about the validity of access needs.

We can foster a culture of access where we all feel connected and expected, where we are able to show up as our full selves without the demand to defend or divulge our trauma. We can create a culture where we are not exhausted or exposed by access labor, where we treat all access needs as valid without verification. We can champion a culture of access that recognizes the politics of disclosure: that many do not have the privilege to declare their disabilities. We can create a culture of access built on the prophetic witness that we all have access needs that deserve to be met.

Whenever my access needs are met, it is like being held by water; my whole body is weightless yet wrapped in buoyancy. It is liberating and light, comforting and calm, and it transforms the trappings of community into a site of care and collective access.[6]

Rather than thinking of access as a checklist, I wonder if we can begin to think of it as a choreography. Sure, there are requirements, regulations, and rules when it comes to access, but ADA is a floor, not a ceiling. It is neither comprehensive nor extensive. Creating a culture of access cannot be found solely in some stuffy old law. Laws alone do not cultivate a culture of access. Policy is not practice. That begins by acknowledging that everyone has access needs and by working as a community to meet those access needs with curiosity and care.

There are set parameters to cultivating access but also movement and interdependence between, around, and above those. It is like a dance. A dynamic, interdependent dance, where we're invited to co-create the moves. Think about anytime "Cha-Cha

6. For more on collective access and the principles of disability justice, check out "10 Principles of Disability Justice," Sins Invalid, accessed December 9, 2025, https://sinsinvalid.org/10-principles-of-disability-justice.

Slide" plays at a party. Each of us are doing the same moves but with different grooves. One hop this time. Right foot, two stomps. Left foot, two stomps. Slide to the left. Access choreography is like that. We get to co-create the dance with one another. Real smooth, let's go to work!

Access choreography is not merely reliant on one person. It invites responsiveness and connectivity instead of sticking to a set of guidelines without fluidity. Fixed yet flexible. It allows for multiple people to co-create for the purpose of co-flourishing. It is messy, slow, and vibrant.

In my experience, the disability community has already developed ways to cultivate a culture of access because we are less attached to the myth of our own self-making. The park and the laundromat are a great example of that disability wisdom in practice. We know that we have access needs. We know that we are human. That allows us to stop pretending that we are God and to get on with the work of supporting one another however we can. I have learned so much from the prophetic witness of my disabled friends about the value of our community in the way we show up, show out, and dance like no one is watching. Real smooth.

In a culture of access, there is no doubting or demonstrating that we are disabled "enough." There are access needs that get to be met. There is no need for staring or glaring, but a common commitment to inviting people to engage in whatever way is most accessible to them that day. Push pops, fidget spinners, signing, stimming, leaving, staying, and swaying are all welcome. Or not showing up at all. There is no expectation of communicating in one way or another but the knowledge that silence is golden (and duct tape is silver). There are many modes of making community: online, in person, and asynchronous, to name a few. There is no ticking clock shaming us to share, or stress to process within a set time frame, because we know that time is a construct.

We know that access is inherently relational. It happens over one bowl of chili at the park and one load of towels at the laundromat at a time. We expect there to be access friction in any community and welcome collective problem-solving to practice a culture of access together. There's not just one person in charge of access. There is no utopia universe where all access needs are met without flexibility. There is community where we collectively prioritize creating a culture of access, one step, stomp, and slide at a time.

One way to put this into practice is to begin a gathering with an access invitation or access check-in. In church speak, we might call this an *invocation*. This is a simple way of setting an intention for the space we co-create, acknowledging that we all have access needs and that we want to be a part of supporting one another's. Inviting everyone to get up, get down, pace, take up space, communicate, and participate in whatever way is accessible that day is just one way that our access needs are anticipated and accepted. We are often made to feel like we're disruptive when using sensory tools in the middle of a service, small group, or sermon. People might give us the side-eye or mean mug. We're often blamed for being the problem. Inviting us up front to show up in whatever way is accessible to us is one way to educate a broader community that we want disabled people here. It acknowledges that access needs shift from day to day and proclaims that no disruption is worth the exclusion of disabled people. It is our way of saying, "You belong here."

How will we know when we have contributed to a culture of access? We will likely start late because time is a construct. Something—or many somethings—will not go as planned because someone is so low on spoons it cuts like a knife. Some folks will leave halfway through. Someone will show up out of the blue. Others will speak up when we plan for quiet. Or need food to follow a certain diet. Furniture will be rearranged. Transportation will be changed. People will sit, stand, roll, sign, stim, and dance their way into co-flourishing. It will be messy and mercurial, and some asks might not feel ideal, but it will be the real deal. Creating a culture of access is not neat and it's never complete, but it is critical to the way we build communities. It is just one way that we practice the prophetic witness of the disability community by ensuring that access is nuanced yet nonnegotiable.

Accessibility is an asset because it allows us to build bonds with more of our neighbors. It allows us to connect with each member of the beloved community. It allows us to acknowledge the fullness of our humanity and dispel the myth that we are robots.

Dream with me for a moment. What if your day was not so full of places to be and things to do that you had to caffeine your way through? What if you gave yourself permission to honor your access needs, whatever they might be on any given day? Disabled people are prophetic because we acknowledge we have access needs, and we have generated expertise in how to collectively meet them. We have so much cultural wealth to share with anyone who would learn.

Disability has been a prophetic catalyst in my life, helping bring clarity to the chaos. There is still chaos, but I think I notice details about the way we build society better because I am disabled. Yet disability cannot be reduced to something as simple as being a good teacher. I am grateful for the way disability has formed my life and my faith, and I also recognize that being disabled is not the sum total of who I am.

We can invite the way that disability disrupts the myths that we have been taught about ourselves and one another. We are so much more than our accolades and accomplishments. Our credentials are not our character. We are taught to scurry onto the hamster wheel of hustle culture, pushing past any internal barriers into the burnout of success. We pretend that we do this out of obligation or ambition, but it is killing us. Literally killing us. We shouldn't have to mask our access needs to fit in, and we don't need to stick to what has been done in the past. What if tradition is really just peer pressure from dead people?

We all have access needs. It's just that most nondisabled people are used to having their access needs met without much fanfare. Inaccessibility denies our humanity. It limits our communities from fully thriving. And not just me. Not just our unhoused neighbors. *All* of us.

What if instead of piling access labor on one another, we supported a culture of access so that everyone could thrive? What if we stopped questioning people's access needs and instead started inviting the way disability disrupts our previous practices and planning? What if we stopped limiting disabled people and recognized the ways disability is valuable to all of us?

As Alice Wong, Mia Mingus, and Sandy Ho remind us, access is love.[7] Creating a culture of access requires that nondisabled people be patient, and it requires that they be kind. It is not something to boast about or roast one another for later. Creating a culture of access is not loud or proud. It always protects disabled people, always trusts disabled people, always hopes that a more accessible world is possible. Creating a culture of access is love.

We can create a culture of access from every boardroom to boardwalk, from every airport to basketball court, from the jail to the hiking trail, from the museum to the Colosseum (which now has an elevator, by the way). We can create a culture of access in every small group and Girl Scout troop, from every classroom to bathroom, and in every mission, ministry, and message. It's a love story, baby, just say yes (to access).

7. Check out the Access Is Love project by Mia Mingus, Alice Wong, and Sandy Ho, "Access Is Love," Disability Visibility Project, February 1, 2019, https://disabilityvisibilityproject.com/2019/02/01/access-is-love.

PRACTICE

By yourself, in a small group, or with a friend, I invite you to think about how we can create a culture of access.

What's an example of an access need? Think about language, practices, the built environment, tactile experiences, food, sensory experiences, the digital environment, pace, structures, and systems. Maybe it's your own access need or one that you are familiar with. Maybe it's one that you learned about in this chapter. I've given a few to start us off:

- Quiet space
- Color contrast
- Wide aisles for Deaf space
-
-

How can we create a culture of access together? What can you do in your community to create a culture of access right now? Your answers can respond to the access needs listed above or be unrelated. Here are some ideas to get you started:

- Offer an access invitation
- Use alt text
-
-

Creating a culture of access happens at the level of community, and we know that creating this culture takes all of us. May these ideas spur us to action, wherever we find ourselves.

6

MY DISABILITY IS POWERFUL

"This has never happened before," the nurse apologizes, the 22-gauge buckling in my forearm. I read the shock on her face before registering the crooked needle crushed by my veins alone. The scrubs tell me not to look, but I always do. I am the only witness to what is done to my bodymind.

The nosy needle is now barbed wire gnawing at my flesh. My nurse's horror is so overwhelming at the buckling that my eyes momentarily avert to her face. I think of myself as Wonder Woman, but I didn't expect that would come with the ability to bend stainless steel. I prod her with this joke. She chuckles a little too candidly, causing the needle to nettle me further. It is worth it just for the laugh.

I am on week two of trying to reset my nervous system, which requires hanging out at the hospital for several weeks in a row. Talk about becoming a new creation. Thursdays are now full of IVs instead of discussion of the "Ivies." I swap out conversations with students for being stabbed by scrubs, sometimes in my arm but most of the time in my spine. I comfort the nurse as she twists the treacherous steel out from my bruised skin and grabs gauze to gag the gushing. Still wearing the bruises from last week, my shy veins are even harder to find. They only make an appearance in a watercolor way, evaporating in the background of my bruises. I needle the nurse that there's a needle-in-a-haystack joke in there somewhere. She doesn't even smirk. I hate to be there when the laughter stops.

It takes two nurses, five tries, and an infrared tool called the Vein Finder™ to get the job done. The procedure has not even started yet, but I have already cemented my status as a medical marvel—my ability to bend metal, a superpower nobody asked for, least of all me. I'd settle for them ironing out my nervous system. For much of my career, students have playfully called me "Professor X," but was I Magneto all along?

Still thinking about the applications of my newfound superpower, I watch them wheel me in for the procedure. I am sure to be funny so the doctors think of me as human. One recent study found that 80 percent of US doctors think disabled people have a poor quality of life, so they won't offer us the same interventions as nondisabled people.[1] Why bother? We're already disabled, or so the thinking goes. In one of my group chats, disabled friends share stories about wearing a fake engagement ring to the doctor's office so the white coats know that someone—anyone—cares about us, loves us. Somehow, I don't think this is what churchy subculture had in mind when they encouraged us to get a ring by spring so we could master in MRS. I guess I shoulda put a faux-gagement ring on it.

My ring is real, but the doctors are so busy asking me about allergies that I don't know if they notice it. Unsure if the doctors clock the rock, I have to make them laugh. Laughter is the best

1. Lisa I. Iezzoni, Sowmya R. Rao, Julie Ressalam, Dragana Bolcic-Jankovic, Nicole D. Agaronnik, Karen Donelan, et al., "Physicians' Perceptions of People with Disability and Their Health Care," *Health Affairs Journal* 40, no. 2 (February 2021), https://doi.org/10.1377/hlthaff.2020.01452.

medicine, and I'm hoping it can be an abatement to ableism for me. No needle can jeopardize my jokes. I'm hoping comedy can endow me with enough humanity in the doctors' minds that they think my life is worth saving if my spinal tap taps into something scary. I know laughter is my ticket to admission to the land of humanity. Their machines infiltrate my body, but they cannot spy the mental calculus it takes for me to be there. Even MRIs, ultrasounds, nerve stimulators, and Vein Finders™ cannot detect the labor of my nervous nervous system. There is no safe house for me at the hospital.

As luck would have it, my anesthesiologist and cane share a name, a pun she immediately gets, having heard all the "Eileen" jokes. (Read: "I lean" because it's a cane. See what I did there?) Their laughter soothes me more than their meds. I inject the room with a few more jokes for good measure. You've heard them all before. There's the one about pain getting on my nerves. And another about stabbing me in the back. I am grateful these medical procedures come with so much punny material. I am grateful these jokes can humanize me to the white coats.

I try not to get in the way as the doctors do their work, prepping and prodding me. My nerves are miscoding messages, like when autocorrect interferes for no particular reason. No, I do *not* want to change "Deaf" to "dead." For duck's sake, autocorrect.

My nerves autocorrect calm to cold, dry to damp, and peace to pain. I feel an icy sensation in my hip but know it's a no-snow zone. My hand feels soaked and soggy, like I just jumped out of my water aerobics class. But when I examine my drenched hand, I find it is not dripping but dry as bone.

Sometimes autocorrect sets my nerves aflame. Fierce, fiery flares devour the left side of my body in sparks and spurts. I didn't start the fire. It was always burning since my nerves were blazing.

And then there's the pain—the autocorrect that gets on my nerves. They send out an SOS: Severe, Obstinate Stabbing. Persistent, pernicious, and prickling, the pain demands to be noticed.

"I'm baaaaaack!" it screeches, clamoring above the chaos. I picture my pain as impeccably well dressed, down to studded stilettos, like a Cruella de Vil type.

She's giving magic, mystique, and mystery. She's electrifying, literally. The pain is often electric, like my nerves are twerking and twitching to a beat no one else knows. I guess they'll keep dancing on their own. It might be alluring if it wasn't so anguishing.

The part that bothers me the most about my nerves autocorrecting isn't the pain or even the strangeness of it all. Why are my nerves suddenly setting fire to the rain? How can I reject the nervous system autocorrect? If my pain happens in a vacuum, and no one hears me scream, is it even real? The part that bothers me the most is that I am not sure how to trust my own bodymind.

Our bodyminds contain so much good data for us. They warn us when something is wrong. They soothe us when something is scary. They steady us when we're traveling on the trauma train. We call their reactions fight, flight, freeze, fawn, or sometimes tend and befriend. We know our bodyminds respond in these ways to protect us.

So many of us have been taught that our disabled bodyminds are bad or sad. We are taught to change for the sake of another's comfort. Nondisabled people love when we have prosthetics, growth hormones, or cochlear implants. Why learn sign language when they can force d/Deaf people to change? Even autocorrect wants Deaf people dead.[2] Nondisabled people love when we come adapted, instead of adapting to our access needs so everyone can thrive. They use tech to leave their ableist nonsense unchecked. As cyborg Jillian Weise says, "They want us shiny and metallic in their image."[3]

Yet we know that our disabled bodyminds are created good. Don't take my word for it. Just ask God. God calls us "very good"

2. Aimee Chou wrote a play about this very thing: *Autocorrect Thinks I'm Dead.*

3. Jillian Weise, "Common Cyborg," *Granta*, September 24, 2018, https://granta.com/common-cyborg.

(Gen. 1:31). God delights in us and rejoices over us (Zeph. 3:17). We are God's masterpiece (Eph. 2:10).

Imagine the awe sparked by sitting in one of Yayoi Kusama's immersive infinity rooms, or in beholding the gouged-out hearts of Frida Kahlo's *The Two Fridas*, the shimmering glint of Gustav Klimt's *The Kiss*, the vibrant hue of Jean-Michel Basquiat's *Boy and Dog in a Johnnypump*, or the swirls of sky in Vincent van Gogh's *Starry Night*. Imagine the emotion evoked by Nina Simone crooning that she's feeling good, Queen asking us to do the fandango, Stevie Wonder's chromatic harmonica in "Isn't She Lovely?" or the emotional journey of Beethoven's symphonies, with the *dun-dun-dun-dun* you can feel in your gut. What a banger.

Imagine the captivating cinematography of Akira Kurosawa's *Throne of Blood*, the sweeping score of *Jurassic Park*, the hand-drawn animation of *Spirited Away*, the watercolor whimsy of *Gris*, or our pure delight in the best *Star Wars* movie ever made, *The Empire Strikes Back*. (Don't come for me.)

These are masterpieces. Triumphs, pleasures, and treasures. Just like us. We are made of the same stuff as each one of these gems. Disabled people are powerful because we are masterpieces. If only we would let our light shine.

It took me a long time to believe that in my bones. I grew up in a household that taught me that everyone was made in the image of God, and I had the audacity to believe it. I knew that people who tried to pray me away subscribed to toxic theology long before I knew the words "theodicy" or "prosperity gospel." But I absorbed some of this corrupt coding along the way from well-meaning ministers and mentors, who taught me that my body was wicked above all else and had the potential to become a chewed-up piece of gum or poop in a brownie, at a moment's notice. Being a disabled woman growing up in purity-culture-era Christianity will do that to you. You're led to believe you're double the trouble, double the sin. My journey to becoming a new creation was an inaccessible path paved with the rubble of shame, insecurity, and ableism, much of it given to me by the church.

Embodying everyone's worst-case scenario does something to you after a while when you're only able to get in through the back door, like no one really wants you around. Cast out by the very people who claim to love you. It took time to excavate the precious jewels in the rubble: that we are image bearers. That our disabled bodyminds are divine. That no powers or principalities can take away from the fact that we are loved.

So for me to not trust my bodymind about what she shares with me is dissociating. I have spent so much time unlearning and relearning my relationship with my bodymind, coaching myself that I am trustworthy, that I have been "fearfully and wonderfully made" (Ps. 139:14). Not if I am "fixed" or fussed over. Right here, right now. My disabled bodymind is wonderfully made, just like those masterpieces.

Sprawled out on a hospital bed with the specter of autocorrect looming in the room, I am still not sure if I can trust my bodymind. That's the part I'm not supposed to say out loud because I'm so focused making a case for why disabled people aren't rejects. Lurking beneath this is the truth that often I don't want to admit, even to myself, that sometimes I cannot rely on my bodymind. Some days, my bodymind autocorrects in ways I wish she would not. Some days, I am agitated, not just with ableism but with autocorrect itself. Some days, I am not sure which pieces of my bodymind I can trust.

I want to share the messy truth of my experience, because I think it is more compelling than a neat lie. The truth will set you free and all that. I want to tell you that disability is powerful, radiant, and divine, while honoring the pieces of my disability that are confusing, complicated, and chaotic.

Disability is not just one thing, and it can't be contained by reductive adages and axioms. Disability is an identity, an experience, a community, and a culture that contains a wide range of physical, mental, cognitive, and sensory experiences. With that comes a variety of ways that disabled people understand our bodyminds and the way we interact with the world around us.

Sometimes disabled people have been forced into narratives of perseverance, resilience, and resistance, and those stories deserve to be told. Sometimes disabled people feel pressured to tell stories purely of pride and positivity to prove that we are worthy of dignity and respect. But mine is a different story: not one strictly of disability positivity or pessimism but a nuance that comes from the wisdom of knowing that life is more complicated than that. I do not want to be grim or glib but genuine.

For me, disability just is. Disability is part of the biodiversity of humanity and a key way that I interact with the world around me. Disability has taught me to savor moments I might otherwise have missed. My disability is at times hard and heavy, not just because of the way society excludes me but because of physical pain that I endure. My disability is murky and muddled, and I do not wish to erase the confounding components of my experience just to tell a simplified story.

I am no suffering servant or pious patient. I am no deity or demon. I am someone who affirms the divinity of disability all the while recognizing how complicated my bodymind behaves. My disability has taught me more about nuance than any class ever could. She shows me what it means to become a new creation and become more like Creator, autocorrecting nerves and all (Col. 3:10). My disabled bodymind has taught me what it means to be human.

In the recovery room, I feel tingly. Spasms are my move. Guessing I am shivering, the needling nurse fetches an itchy blanket that I appreciate but don't need. I am at the nerve disco inferno. Every ninety seconds or so, my nerves do the electric slide. I breathe in gratitude for my bodymind for telling me what is going on, even if it's in a dead dance dialect I can't yet decipher. *You can't see it! It's electric!* I clock the second hand slowly grazing each number on the wall to steady myself. With each passing tick, I breathe in and out, slowly, spasm-y.

The left side of my body warms as if someone has cloaked me in a cozy cloud. It's like in a cartoon, when a storm cloud follows only Eeyore. Except the cloud isn't dark and stormy. It kindles with all the warmth of a cuppa. Thanks for noticing me. The puffy, fluffy clouds drift down my left thigh, knee, and ankle, until I can feel their heat externally. Outside, there is still snow on the ground, but fire is coursing through my veins. So much fire it makes a dragon wanna retire. My left side is six degrees toastier to the touch. I've never felt anything like it. Burn, baby, burn!

Much of my high school years were spent warding off "threats" of amputation because of a lack of circulation. My left leg was more blue than body, my toes stuck together like glue. No wiggle room for them. Doctors wanted to Frankenstein a bodymind that was shinier and less spasm-y. I wasn't a hothead; I was a cold foot. My left side, one cool cat, always at least 15 degrees colder than the right. So many hours were spent learning to raise my temperature as I would watch on the monitors as the numbers climbed, willing it to get to 90 degrees Fahrenheit before the end of the session. I've never been described as "warm" before.

Anticipating news in the waiting room, my husband texts me to check in, and I respond with hot takes as heat radiates from my reawakened leg. Somehow this isn't what he had in mind when I said we'd be sending "steamy texts." As we pass by the snowcapped trees on the drive home, we marvel at the Thursday Night Fever becoming the new jig of my leg. The heat is visible. My left leg is at least four shades warmer than my right, her warmth unable to be contained by flesh and bone alone.

My disabled bodymind resets, nerve by nerve. What does it feel like? It's like moving through molasses with the slow-mo filter on. I can think of no better way to describe the sensation of watching my decrepit nerves come back to life than the valley of dry bones. As Ezekiel gazed at the valley, "there was a noise, a rattling, and the bones came together, bone to its bone. I looked, and there were sinews on them, and flesh had come upon them, and skin had covered them; but there was no breath in them" (37:7–9).

Something I love about the valley of dry bones is how gnarly it all is. It feels true to my experience of disability: to linger in the languish a little longer before rushing ahead to the resurrection; to allow the grimy, slimy bones to creak and crack beneath the earth; to hang out in graveyards long enough to be soiled by their soil. The valley of dry bones is gruesome and grotesque. Limbs withering, sinews slithering, and tendons shivering to twist and twiddle together. Severed body parts that were once declared "ashes to ashes, dust to dust," resurrecting once more.

When we say that we want to "practice resurrection," we sometimes skip ahead to the end of the story, superimposing a triumphant narrative on the whole thing. But resurrection always comes by way of death. It isn't an erasure of everything preceding it. The way resurrection has unfolded in my life has been through a series of deaths—some minor, some major—but all painful. The death of what I can do on Thursday afternoons, of life's expected timeline, of a mythology of self, and of needs left unmet. The road to resurrection has been paved with a series of deaths: gory graveyards stacked with the ashes of my expectations, hopes, and dreams.

There was no noise, but I did feel my nervous system rattling, spasming, jerking back to life. I suppose my neuropathways are now smooth sailing for my nerves, traveling on the highway between my head and my heels. The valley of dry nerves has been brought back to life in a frigid hospital room one January afternoon through jokes and jabs. It's less *Dawn of the Dead* and more *Kill Bill*. It's the only way I know how to practice resurrection: by way of death. Ashes to ashes, dust to dust.

Some days, my nerves autocorrect once more. I wonder how I can get through another round of nerve resurrection roulette.

I feel like a sarcophagus masquerading as a meat sack. I wonder if my bones will buckle under the pressure of pursuing resurrection. Can these bones live? Some days, I want my nerves to stop getting on my last nerve. Yet this I call to mind, and therefore I have hope: Even the most desolate areas of our lives can be brought back to life. Nothing is beyond repair. No one is beyond redemption. In fact, we are all masterpieces.

Holding onto hope that our lives are worth it, even when no one else dares to care, is no easy task. It takes more than I want to give. Yet time and again, that has been my experience with being a disabled masterpiece. Disability can demonstrate the divine to us, if only we have the grit to receive its gruesome reality. What makes me powerful isn't that my nerves autocorrect or that I can bend metal like Magneto. What makes me powerful is that I know the truth: We are divine, and that doesn't mean we are shielded from death. We are not the "before" picture of a prayer makeover or the symbol of sin used to guilt others into repenting. We are not chewed-up pieces of gum or bathroom brownies. Disabled people are a vibrant, radiant, powerful part of the beloved community, and we have much to teach the church about what it means to be human. Disabled people are masterpieces.

I will keep rebelling against anyone who tells me otherwise. Why? Rebellions are built on hope. Something that we learned from *Rogue One*, the *actual* best *Star Wars* movie ever made. (Don't come for me.)

Since this hospital stint, my nerves continue to autocorrect. I am not sure if I can trust my bodymind, but I practice listening to her anyway. I try to honor her nerve disco dance, even when I don't understand all the moves. Being disabled has developed a muscle that I might not otherwise have: one that makes me know that not everything is linear, neat, or complete. One that recognizes that my bodymind is too much of a messy masterpiece to ever be contained. One that has made peace with uncertainty, and friends with flexibility.

The truth is I am not concerned about whether my leg will die again because I have survived that. I am made of stronger stuff than blood and bone. The thing about practicing resurrection is that you end up spending a lot of time in graveyards. Death is the concern of empires, not of resurrection people. Declaring power over death is alluring in a spiritual bypassing kind of way, but in my experience, death and pain sure do sting. Mine is not to profess that my reawakened leg was "worth" the pain, or even whether the procedures "worked" as promised. I don't have a metric for such maxims. I am more interested in proclaiming that my life is worth living—in, with, and through the pain. I am not hoping for medical magic but a transformation by the truth: Uncomplicated and unexamined platitudes are dressed up as theology.

We are not nearly as powerful as our tidy theologies like to pretend we are. We are fickle, fragile, and frail. Our very being rests on a breath. Declaring that we are powerful isn't about affirming that we are above all the emotions and experiences of humanity but delving into them—nerve first and spine deep—and declaring with our bodyminds that our lives are worth living, even when parts of us are dying.

Sometimes I wonder how many disabled people haven't been allowed to grow up as ourselves. We grow up playing an expected version of ourselves that sacrifices authenticity to minimize prejudice and pain. We become cardboard cutouts of our characters. For me, that meant masking instead of grasping the way that the very act of performing a painless facade was fatiguing. Trauma twists us into a living memorial to ourselves, reliving the most painful parts of our pasts in each new era. But I don't want my life to be a memorial or a maxim; I want my life to be lived, breathed, and felt—even when what I feel is pain.

Lying on the sterile crinkling paper in yet another hospital room, I try to disentangle the pieces of myself that are real and the ones that are reactive; the wisecracks from wisdom; the armor from authenticity. I try to untwine the threads of myself that I've woven together like chain mail as protection. I try to scrap my shields and sit in my own serpentine sincerity. It is slippery and unsettling, and it is sacred.

The truth is, my disabled bodymind is messy, miraculous, mercurial, and mundane. I am grateful for my disabled bodymind, and yet there are parts of her I am still learning how to understand. I might say the same of faith.

When I say that disabled people are powerful, I mean that we reveal what is true about all of us, that there is no hierarchy of humanity, that life is desolate and delightful, that there are no limits on the divine. Nothing we produce or practice can add to or take away from that. We are from ashes, and to ashes we will one day return. We are powerful because with every joke and jab, we boldly proclaim that disabled people are messy masterpieces. The hope of my life is not to transcend the ashes but to transform them. I am my most powerful when I am honest about my limits and I can revel in my humanness.

I grip the chilly rail of the hospital bed as I remind myself that my disabled bodymind is powerful, one gem that I excavate from the ashes of expectation.

But do you not know what Creator can do with just a little bit of ash?

PRACTICE

Doctors are obsessed with pain charts. What if we could reclaim the pain chart to focus on the sacredness of our bodyminds? Blessing our bodyminds does not erase the torment and trauma many of us have and continue to experience. Instead, this practice invites us to consider how our bodyminds are already magnificent, messy masterpieces.

On a figure below that you connect to, draw:

/ / / /	Places that you are grateful for
XXXX	Places that radiate the divine
OOOO	Places that take care of you
====	Places that are trustworthy
++++	Places that you want to bless

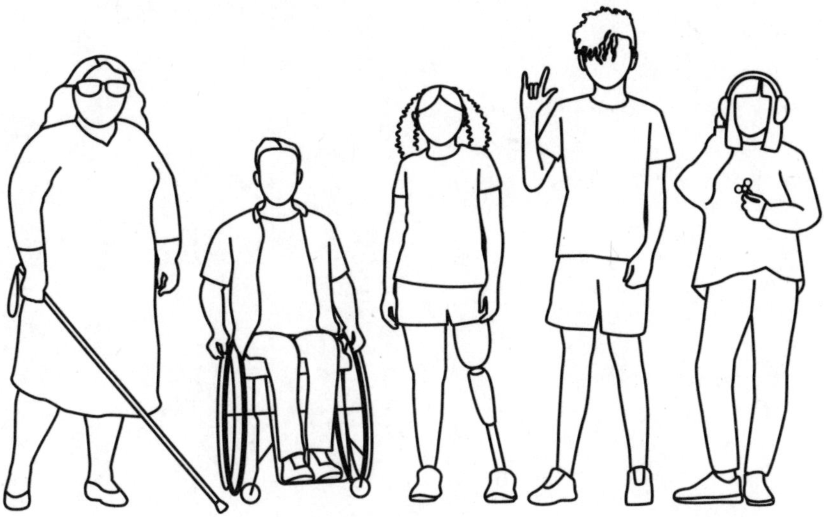

7

MY DISABILITY IS A SACRED LAMENT

It's not until the third cotton ball filled with my blood passes under my nose that I realize I am in surgery. It wasn't when the resident injected anesthetic into my face. Or when the surgeon slashed a chunk of my cheek out with a scalpel. Or when I waited there, alone in a sterile room, unsure of what to do with my arms, for three rounds of this stabbing, numbing, cutting routine. It was when the surgeons were trying to halt the hemorrhage and the blood-soaked cotton grazed my nose. Four hours, fifteen stitches, and one skin graft later, I am cancer free.

In the doctor's office, I am all ages at once. I float in and out of memories of other sterile rooms full of different white coats but the same load-bearing traumas.

The nurse shoves consent forms on my lap, and suddenly I am eleven again, eavesdropping as my doctors and parents argue over my best course of treatment, trying to understand what the word "amputation" means. It is hard to comprehend consent when I legally don't have it. After all, it's just my bodymind.

I draw circles with my fingers on the medical crepe paper as I wait for the lab results to confirm the cancer is gone. I am fourteen again, doodling shapes on a different bed laced with the same crispy covering as my dad gets kicked out after telling the neurologist not to blame my pain solely on me being a teenage girl. I've never seen my dad expelled out of anywhere. He's what you'd call stoic. I don't yet know what the word "psychiatric" means, but the emotion of it is projected onto my dad's face.

Now, as they bandage my face, the resident instructs me on a lengthy list of post-op no-no's. There are the obvious ones of no heavy lifting or hard foods, but the one that bothers me the most is no smiling or laughing for two weeks. Abruptly, I am thirteen again, watching the pharmacist's soft smile fade while he ushers me to the side of the blood pressure cuff and whispers to my mum, her face veiled in tears. Eavesdropping, I scribble "fen-tylenol" on my palm, not knowing why a drug that sounds like Tylenol's fencing cousin would make my mum weep.

From the current hospital bed, I ask the surgeon where I'll fall on the scale of facial scars from Harry Potter to Scarface, and he promises me I'll still be beautiful. I hate myself for feeling relief.

I am transported to a different hospital, with a different surgeon, reassuring me I'll look good in a bikini. On that hospital visit, the doctors brush off my abdominal agony while my appendix ruptures inside of me. I almost died because they didn't believe my pain, but at least my body is beach ready. A bikini is the furthest thing from my mind while covered in iodine and freshly stitched incisions that almost *didn't* save my life.

Maybe that's why it took me so long to recognize that I was in surgery, downplaying my pain even to myself. I don't want to cause a scene, to be branded hysterical again. I don't want to *be* a pain when I am in pain. I want to get an A+ in being in pain, even if that nonsense doesn't make the grade.

When the doctor called to tell me it was cancer, she was so apologetic, her words more like a gentle breeze than a gusty wind.

"It's not *your* fault," I reassured her, desperately wanting to ease her distress, not wanting to be the cause of her discomfort when explaining my pain. I played the role of the patient patient perfectly.

It wasn't until later that I realized *she's* not the one I wanted an apology from. It's the doctor who told me it was *just* my period when my ovaries required surgery. It's the doctor who told me it was *just* the flu when my appendix burst. It's the doctors—dozens of them, names and faces and white coats a blur—who told me I was faking it before I was diagnosed with a rare nerve condition. I was just a girl. It's easier to brand me a problem than listen to my pain.

And it's me, for believing them for so long. For concealing my pain lest it be dismissed or doubted again. For using degrees to endow myself with the humanity they strip away from me because I am disabled. I am all alone in yet another hospital room, praying for someone to believe me, to treat me like my life is worth living. I lament that I am here again, with only the wounds no one can witness to carry my woes.

I am not that eleven-year-old girl anymore, wondering what medical words mean. I now teach students about big ideas. I've collected degrees in words and word play, hoping my wisdom will procure me adequate medical care—casually dropping my résumé to each white coat in hopes that they will believe me, a disabled woman, about my pain. The letters after my name are the only language they speak.

I am not that eleven-year-old girl anymore, but she still comes with me to doctor's appointments. She hovers in the room, reminding me that my pain is real and that I can survive this.

And some days, I almost believe her. Maybe one day, doctors will too.

We already know that doctors dismiss women's pain. Study after study confirms that Black women in particular are more likely to receive anti-anxiety medication or outright discharge when presenting pain in the emergency room.[1] What's the data for disabled women, you ask? I wish I could tell you. We don't have the stats, because medicine doesn't care about us enough to study that. We *do* know that 80 percent of doctors believe that disabled people have a poor quality of life and therefore don't offer the same interventions to us as they do to nondisabled people.[2] I guess they forgot about their foremost oath: First, do no harm.

Our pain is dismissed whenever we have the courage to voice it. Our bodies reduced to bikini bods or "beautiful" scar-faces whenever we have the nerve to notice or name our pain. The medical-industrial complex is still treating us like frightened eleven-year-olds who don't have consent over our own bodyminds. And at every phase, the church has been there, telling me "Everything happens for a reason" and "God wouldn't give you more than you can handle."

How many women and young girls are there, knowing their pain will not be believed by their doctors or pastors? How many women and girls downplay their destruction on the daily?

"God is in control," people coo. There is little space to lament in communities who would rather use thought-terminating clichés than practice what they preach. There is no clapback to this. No answer that is big enough to counter this cliché. It is designed as a shutdown. If you try to say, "Hey, that's not cool" because it spiritually bypasses real pain, it can easily turn into a theological debate. If you try to point out that lamenting is part of the church's heritage and history, you get called a heretic. There is no space for humanity in a community that is more interested in upholding

1. Maureen Salamon, "The Dangerous Dismissal of Women's Pain," *Harvard Health*, July 1, 2025, https://www.health.harvard.edu/pain/the-dangerous-dismissal-of-womens-pain.

2. Lisa I. Iezzoni, Sowmya R. Rao, Julie Ressalam, Dragana Bolcic-Jankovic, Nicole D. Agaronnik, Karen Donelan, et al., "Physicians' Perceptions of People with Disability and Their Health Care," *Health Affairs Journal* 40, no. 2 (February 2021), https://doi.org/10.1377/hlthaff.2020.01452.

its toxic positivity than pursuing authentic connectivity.[3] Good vibes are great, but when they are all we can tolerate, it leaves no space for the grime and grit of life. Have they ever met the Man of Sorrows?

Spaces that preach positivity above all else are exhausting. Lament is terrifying to those who subscribe to such views. Emotions scare them. How long, O Lord, must we suffer the silencing of our pain?

My disability has a way of cultivating lament, because many Christian communities have decided to dismiss us. I lament that I am so accustomed to animosity and apathy about my agony that it has become anticipated—average, even. But it should be neither accepted nor expected. The real lament about disability isn't our bodyminds or the way we show up in the world; it's the way the world shows up for us. It's the way the church doesn't show up for us at all. How long, O Lord?

"Will you come hold my hand while I die?" she asked, as if inviting me to dinner rather than a death.

My friend Sharon and I initially bonded over our shared medical trauma, a common pastime among chronically ill and disabled folks. We both knew what it was like for doctors to dismiss us, for our pain to not be "real" to the white coats, and we held space for one another to share it without shame or shutdown.

Sharon wanted to die surrounded by people who know her as more than a medical case file, in the comfort of her own home. She had lived there for less than a year with mismatched, donated furniture with too many traces of the tastes of previous tenants. She only qualified for it because she was less than six months away

3. Andrew Pulrang, "People with Disabilities Have a Complicated Relationship with 'Positivity,'" *Forbes*, July 22, 2021, https://www.forbes.com/sites/andrewpulrang/2021/06/22/people-with-disabilities-have-a-complicated-relationship-with-positivity.

from death. It turns out lung cancer was the only key to unlocking housing for this pediatric nurse who called her Nissan Maxima home after "medical bankruptcy" came knocking.

When I first met Sharon at the park, she was sifting through a box of bras that someone donated to folks experiencing homelessness. As we made self-conscious small talk, she loudly voiced her candid assessment of each intimate—violet lace, black T-shirt, a padded scarlet number that raised her eyebrows—saying, "Oooh, too fancy!" or "NO!" With each bra, the pretense of politeness dwindled between us. By the time she reached the bottom of the box, we were fast friends, two spoonies who knew how to laugh.[4]

That sort of "doesn't make sense but just go with it" vibe is the hallmark of our community. There's that one time some random woman at the laundromat chipped in ten dollars after noticing we were a community with mostly unhoused folks the first Sunday of every month. You would have thought it had Benjamin's face on it, the delight it drew out of our friends. "Wow, people just *give* you folks money," one of them teased us for weeks to come. There's that other time we pushed a truck—a monster of an F-150—for half a mile so one of our friends wouldn't get a sixty-dollar parking ticket. Every unexpected expense is an emergency when you don't have the luxury of not sweating the small stuff.

We've painted on patios and celebrated holidays together, each year in a different location after being kicked out, but always with plenty of carols and cheer. Life among our friends experiencing homelessness has been a string of wild and wacky stories—like the night a coyote licked one of our friend's toes. I've learned to just show up, even when it doesn't fully make sense.

So Sharon's email asking me to hold her hand while she died wasn't exactly unexpected—I had come to expect the unexpected in my years in the disability community—but it still wrung out my

4. To learn about spoon theory, check out Christine Miserandino, "The Spoon Theory," in *Beginning with Disability: A Primer*, ed. Lennard J. Davis (Routledge, 2017), 174–78.

lungs like a sponge. *Breathe*, I coached myself, reading the details of her date with death, aware of the irony of my lungs tightening up at this request from my friend with lung cancer. I know it is cheaper to die than to be disabled, but it didn't stop me from lamenting that fact all the same. I said I would hold her hand, but in the end, death killed her plans to go to her final home at home.

She was rushed to the hospital with difficulty breathing. The hospice nurse called me from the ambulance, advising me to "make arrangements," which is medical speak for imminent death. It was near the beginning of the Covid closures, when most hospitals were on lockdown. The beds were full but the hallways were empty. Sharon was sedated, but I was the one who felt like a zombie, wandering through the vacant halls as if I were wading against the waves with skinny jeans on.

She didn't speak with words, but her eyes told me she knew my voice, and her knowing smirk reassured me that she was with me behind the machine helping her breathe. I held my phone to her ear for her brother to say goodbye. Me, the secretary to his grief. Hovering next to death, I felt the gravity of knowing this would be the last time I would be with her and wanted to make sure I said something meaningful for her final journey.

I told her how much she was loved and how we'd take care of her wishes, right down to the detailed list of who gets her beat-up recliner (Ava) and the janky space heater she overused (Uzi). Neither of us knew it then, but the biggest hit at the giveaway of her stuff would turn out to be a twelve-pack of single-ply—a golden ticket in those early days of Covid. I can still feel the excitement from one of our newly housed disabled veterans, like a kid on Christmas morning, in a pitch reserved for dogs and dolphins. "Look at this!" Elena squealed from the linoleum bathroom, the clank of her cane the beat to the melody of her joy. "TP! Twelve whole rolls!" Laughter erupted at the silliness of it all. How ecstatic we were with the pure joy that even toilet paper can bring when every expense is expensive.

There in the hospital room, I didn't know any of this yet, but I knew Sharon. I knew how clever and crafty she was. I knew that she wanted her life to be "useful" to people above all else. So I told her that we would take care of it all, and that her life would be useful, since that's what I knew she needed. At the time, I thought I was saying it for her. I now realize it was also for me. I'm still not sure about praising the utility of a life. She squeezed my hand. Belabored and trembling, as though the last ounces of life were spilled on that squeeze. Guess she got to hold my hand while dying after all. It just wasn't at home how she'd imagined.

The next time I went to the hospital was to collect her belongings. Some personal papers, her worn out Crocs, and a donated fuchsia T-shirt that still smelled like the green soap she got at the 99-cent store. That, and a long list of logistics to do after someone dies. She had seventeen dollars and a raggedy recliner to her name.

The cheapest cremation package was $720, including a fog-gray plastic urn that the plucky mortician, à la Janet from *The Good Place*, stressed was *temporary*. "A steal," he'd tried to convince us, when Sharon and I met there one clammy Tuesday at dusk. It costs a lot to live when you are forced into poverty, and it costs a lot to die.

It wasn't until the next Saturday while cleaning out her home that I found the envelope. It wasn't with her old nurse's badge or by the photographs of her late mother, or even with the stack of pink bills on her foldaway table we got from the Salvation Army. It was stuffed in the bottom of her underwear drawer, where no one else would think to look. Ours was a friendship forged over intimates. In my experience, there is a unique bond that spoonies have that the rest of the world doesn't fully understand. Little is off limits when you finally meet someone who speaks the language of your disabled bodymind.

The envelope bulged with small bills she'd set aside each month. It wasn't much, but she had started saving what she could to pay for her final home even when she didn't have one of her own.

Sitting on the chair with Ava's name on it (literally, Sharon stuck a Post-it on the recliner so no one would steal it for themselves), I counted out the cash and let my mind wander back to the time I gave Sharon a pixie cut right after she started chemo. She didn't want the uncertainty of waiting for her hair to fall out in clumps, so one Sunday afternoon we got out the scissors and some courage. "Make me look like Andrew," she'd jokingly bossed me around, relishing the makeover moment. It wasn't that she cared about how she looked or even that she wanted to be pampered so much as she wanted to take charge of her own life, a life that had stripped her of so much agency. The haircut was a mechanism for reclaiming her story—stolen when disabled and unhoused—from the snatches of stigma.

That's exactly what she did with her expenses, skipping meals to make ends meet, sweating it out without air conditioning so she could afford to be cremated, choosing between a funeral and food when ends couldn't stretch far enough. She didn't want to be a burden. She didn't want to cost anyone, she told me one breezy afternoon at her favorite park, despite my assurances to the contrary. Sharon was thrifty and thoughtful to her final breath, but I wish she didn't need to be. How long, O, Lord, must our beloveds be forsaken?

We held her service at the park, not the one where she used to live but the one with the lake, where the ducks paddle their worries away and geese steal bread from unsuspecting toddlers waddling too close to the water. We read her beloved Ralph Waldo Emerson poem while nibbling on her favorite Heath cookies. She loved the birds, the grassy nook, the surly squirrels frolicking as they snatched scraps before scampering away. She would sit and watch them on days when she felt hopeless, she told me once. It helped her feel like there was room to breathe.

It has been over six years since we said goodbye to Sharon. Some days I am still haunted when I visit the park. I think about how she brought so much life into the world, first as a pediatric nurse and later at the park to me and to friends who were unhoused. So much abundant life that we lived together. I think about how she deserved better, how even a couple hundred extra bucks each month would have given her the freedom not to make dire decisions worthy of an apocalyptic novel (food or funeral), how it would have allowed her to exhale after holding her breath for so long. I think about how many other Sharons there are who I know and love, who live in the park, and I feel hopeless.

And then I catch a glimpse of a duck, quacking and shuffling, and I remember how much Sharon liked it here. And just for a fleeting moment, I feel like I can breathe.[5]

We live in a world that would rather see disabled people dead than divine. I lament that this is the case. I wonder how Sharon's life would have been different if her access to housing and health care had not been stripped away. I wonder what would have been different if the church had been church to her. I lament that she did not have what many of us take for granted. I lament that she is not the only disabled, unhoused friend I have buried.

Some of us have been cajoled into hiding aspects of ourselves that we've been taught the church can't handle. We've been sold a sack of lies that we are too messy or muddled for God. Nothing could be further from the truth.

God is big enough to hold our anger, our outrage, and our horror at injustice. I find it meaningful that the psalmists write more psalms of lament than any other kind. Lament is not a pit stop along the road to redemption that you have to repent for later.

5. Some of this previously appeared in Amy Kenny, "When Breath Isn't Enough," *The Audacity*, September 15, 2021, https://audacity.substack.com/p/when-breath-isnt-enough-by-amy-kenny.

Lament is often the destination. God hasn't done what the psalmists think God ought to do, and so they lament. People who claim to follow God have betrayed God's beloveds, and so they lament. Loudly, unapologetically. May we do the same.

In many of the psalms, there is no resolution or change in circumstance. There is authentic anger and wholesome woe called out to Creator. Lament is about sharing the fullness of our human experience. And that human experience includes weeping, wailing, and flailing.

Lament is loyalty. We don't waste our breath on something we don't care about. Lament is not detached, distant, or devoid of faith. Lament is some of the most faithful feelings we can offer in the face of injustice. Lament is a way to echo Jesus on the cross, wailing, "My God, my God, why have you forsaken us?" Lament is holy. As Soong-Chan Rah reminds us, "the loss of lament in the American church reflects a serious theological deficiency."[6] Church, I find your lack of faith disturbing.

Perhaps some of us have grown up in a tradition where lament is not what you're "supposed" to say at church. We are quick to chide ourselves for thinking all the bad things, wondering if we are "losing" our faith for daring to grieve. As though faith comes with a reliable road map.

Grief—the internal experience that lament often cries out—is genuine. It allows us to connect with the deepest parts of ourselves that long for more. Grief is a portal of possibility. Jesus is well acquainted with grief. In Scripture, grief and lament are central components to living a faithful life. In fact, Lisa Sharon Harper teaches us that the healing power of lament is required for shalom.[7]

Christian communities have a long tradition of lament, one that complicates overly rational understandings of faith. In the

6. Soong-Chan Rah, *Prophetic Lament: A Call for Justice in Troubled Times* (InterVarsity, 2015), 24.

7. Lisa Sharon Harper, *The Very Good Gospel: How Everything Wrong Can Be Made Right* (WaterBrook, 2020), 100.

Scriptures, faith is not simply some sensible statement about God. It is trusting God with our entire selves—even the deepest wrath that we are embarrassed to admit we feel.

I can think of nothing more sacred than lamenting that image bearers are cast aside and discarded and that the church is often the place where this happens. Lament is not a failure of faith but an act of faith. We wonder what God is even doing. We wonder why the church is complicit. We feel isolated and indignant at the injustice. We cry out to the God who sees, knowing that our lament is not in vain, because God keeps a record of our tears. We cry out to the God who sees when no one else does.

Lament is love. Love big enough to hold all of the messy, mixed-up feelings that we have about God and faith. Love that doesn't carry shame but names us worthy of dignity because we are divine.

Lament is longing. Longing for a new world where we can all thrive. One without so much injustice everywhere we turn. One where our friends don't die because they are disabled and unhoused. One where our pain is not dismissed or doubted. One where image bearers don't need to convince Christians of their humanity.

In my experience, disabled people can teach the church how to lament. We are asked to honor a system that hasn't honored us. We know what it is to be rejected and dejected. We know how to take our trauma and transform it. We know how to nurture a community of care that some might call a church.

The purpose of lamenting is to yearn for a new world. I know grief is a type of time travel. I wonder if hope can be too. When I lament, it is because I hope against hope that we will not have to suffer this injustice any longer. It is a prophetic act that allows us to acknowledge the inequities of this world and to imagine how we can co-create another one. It is an act of ushering in heaven on earth. It is just one way that we participate in creating shalom with the community of creation. As Randy Woodley shows, shalom "is active and engaged, going far beyond the mere absence of conflict.

A fuller understanding of shalom is the key to the door that can lead us to a whole new way of living in the world."[8] We already have that key, and lament can help us unlock a new world together.

If you find yourself disconnected from lament, it might be time to schedule a meeting with yourself. Have you fooled yourself into fawning the false god of numbing your emotions as a source of strength? Repression is not reverence. Are you disconnected from the experience of those in our communities who are suffering from the dehumanizing effects of indifference? Disassociation is not devotion.

I lament that disabled women are not believed in medical settings. I lament that image bearers are discarded and dying on the streets. I lament that many people think disabled people are defective instead of divine. Perhaps most of all, I lament that the church is often first in line in being a place of dismissal and derision. I lament because I know that it does not have to be this way.

We cannot live in the world we want to co-create if we do not begin to imagine it. Lament can be the first phase of creating that new world together, where we can all co-flourish. Once you begin to introduce yourself to a version of yourself that doesn't have to participate in your own masking, you begin to imagine that a different world is not only possible, it is probable.

As Arundhati Roy says, "It is already here. With our art, our music, our literature, our stubbornness, our joy, our brilliance, our sheer relentlessness—and our ability to tell our own stories. Stories that are different from the ones we're being brainwashed to believe. Another world is not only possible, she is on her way. On a quiet day, I can hear her breathing."[9]

8. Randy Woodley, *Shalom and the Community of Creation: An Indigenous Vision* (Eerdmans, 2012), 10.

9. Arundhati Roy, *War Talk* (South End, 2003), 75.

PRACTICE

We have a faithful tradition of sacred lament. Rewrite a lament from your perspective. This might be lamenting the ableism you have experienced or witnessed. Injustice abounds. Lament is not merely complaining or dwelling on a negative experience but a way to turn to God with our anger, hurt, and yearning for a more just world. Here is an example inspired by the psalms:

> How long, O Lord, will we forget disabled people?
> How long must I wrestle with the torment of nondisabled ignorance?
> Scorned by everyone, friend to no one.
> I cry out day and night, but there is no answer.
> My beaten body can no longer wail; my eyes are dry from weeping.
> I am bereft.

Your turn. You might begin with: "How long, O Lord, _____?"

Not vibing? Check out Psalm 13, 22, or 88 for inspiration.

8

MY DISABILITY IS VALUABLE

"I was just trying to *help*," he huffs, after I asked him not to throw trash in my mobility scooter. "Helping" is his rubbish reason for treating Diana's basket as a bin. He mutters how I looked like I needed help, as if that allows him the right to trash me.

"I don't need your trash," I snap, before he finally backs off, arms raised, eyes rolled to the back of his shaking head. Not the best trash talk on my part, but I have had enough of being treated like garbage. I think about giving him the full Kevin McCallister: "I'm gonna give you to the count of ten, to get your ugly, no-good trash off my property, before I pump your guts full of lead!" But I think better of being so cheeky when trying to turn the other cheek. My clear boundary is enough for him to know I won't accept this trashing.

People think that my wheels whelp, "Help, I need somebody! Anybody!" Newsflash: I don't need uninvited help. I am not refusing unsolicited assistance out of pride or to be snide. (I didn't *actually* go Kevin McCallister on the guy. I just wanted him to go home alone.)

I gladly ask and task supporters every day. Yet, so-called helping from untaught and unsought strangers often does more harm than good. Helping often hurts.

Take the Uber driver who is so busy trying to help get me into the car that he becomes a pain in the butt. Literally. He tumbles out of his Toyota Sienna, right onto his backside. Three feet down and nothing to catch him but the road. It looks like it hurts like a bitumen. He is still wiping his asphalt when he drives off, too butt-hurt to take me and my friend after causing a scene in the name of being a saint.

Take the disastrous door opener, who not only upholds an armpit underpass for me to wade through a waft of BO, but also ends up hitting me with the door I didn't need help opening. Or the self-selected bellhop, who grabs my bag without so much as a wink, making me think I am being mugged. Or the pushy pusher, who tries to push my electric wheels for some unknown reason. My wheels have more horsepower than his arms and more stamina than his legs. It makes no sense to push Diana, Princess of the My-Scootra. In fact, pushing often messes with her brakes, so shove off. Walkies are so weird sometimes.

It's the same thing that happens before I go out to eat. I call ahead to make sure the restaurant is accessible enough for my three-wheeled seat.

"Yes, *of course* we are accessible!" a reassuring voice beams back, almost proud of their ability to follow a federal law that is over thirty-five years old. Almost flabbergasted that someone dared to ask. "Our bathroom is just up one small stair. It's *very* negligible."

Negligible? Whenever it comes to wheels, no stair—no matter how tiny or shiny—is negligible. If only there were a series of guidelines determining what "wheelchair accessible" means. Oh, wait. There are. Some folks just don't want to follow them. Pretending stairs are accessible is not helpful; it's harmful.

Helping is not needed or conceded from anyone who thinks they can out-push electric wheels or thinks it's better to lie about access than admit the truth of inaccessibility. They are just spinning their wheels, but I am the one who has to deal with their ableist nonsense. In all of these examples, I directly and explicitly told the harmful helper that I did not need their "help." I even greased the wheels by thanking them for caring. I directed them head-on, but hands-off. In situations like these, I must remain passionate, yet poised; consistent, yet calm; powerful, yet polite. It is a never-ending plight. My words do little to assuage the harmful helper. They think they know best, and they are not afraid to say it.

Never mind that I know Diana (wheels). I know what she hates (being pushed), and how she likes to carry my bag on her arm like freight. I know how high is too steep (2 inches) and why she beep beeps (trying to move in neutral). I know how much space we need to turn (33 inches) and how quickly her wheels burn (10 miles). She doesn't want to climb every mountain and she's not afraid to beep about it. Beeps are not just the sound of her music, but the rhythm of a few of her least favorite things. When the brake bites, when the throttle stings, when she's feeling sad, she simply beeps her least favorite things, so then I don't get so mad. Five beeps for the brake, seven when the throttle has flaked, and eight when the motor is not great. I like to think she has a potty mouth with how much bleeping she does. I know my wheels and what I need help with. And I *never* need help with someone trashing me.

"I was just trying to help!" harmful helpers moan and groan on repeat, as if that excuses hitting, pushing, or mugging someone. I hope I don't have to tell you: This help is not helpful. In fact, it's typically called "assault." It hurts, emotionally and physically. I have been knocked in the head and shoulder checked, and have come away with bruised knees and trampled toes, all from harmful helpers. This is not the version of head, shoulders, knees, and toes that Diana and I want to be singing.

While this happens *to* me, it's not really about me. Harmful helpers are telling on themselves. They reveal the dreary theory that disabled people are utterly helpless and in constant need of unsolicited support. Their behavior conceals arrogance in altruism, convincing both me and the harmful helpful that they know what is best, despite my explicit protests. Somewhere deep down, perhaps even subconsciously, they think they are better than a disabled woman, because they can only act out a script that casts themselves as superior saint and me as suffering subservient. Their behavior inadvertently showcases how valuable disability is in disrupting someone's sense of self.

Many of us have been taught the core lie that nondisabled people are holier or higher on the hierarchy of humanity. There is no such ladder when it comes to dignity and worth. We are all divine. Some of us are just used to it.

If someone is still unconvinced, I wonder if you would grab a stranger's bag without asking if that someone was *not* a disabled woman. I wonder if you would throw trash on a nondisabled man. Literal trash. Not in a lighthearted way like the internet ribbing us Aussies for saying "naur." Or when my Gen Z students joke that I was born in the 1900s. He threw wadded up trash at me! Clearly, I'm still not over it.

It is not that I am above help. I am above being assaulted every time I go out in public. I am above my consent being contradicted. I am above strangers thinking I am not a full human solely because I look at the world from below.

If you're wondering how to be an ally to disabled people, ask us. Offer help, sure. But be open to us refusing it without explanation. Be open to learning from disabled folks when we say we know how and when we need help, if we need help at all. Be open to us saying no, even when you *think* you know best. "Naur" is a complete sentence. Be open to the fact that we are fully human and capable of consent.

It's funny to me that nondisabled people are invested in pushing us, because this is something that doesn't happen when I am with other disabled people. When a friend who uses a manual wheelchair gets tired, she doesn't ask someone to push her. She asks me for a tow. She holds the back of my mobility scooter and we both glide with ease, our wheelchair train becoming an interdependent cruise across the terrain.

Walking isn't desired in these moments. Walking isn't the picture of strength or success. It's wholly unnecessary for us. We don't have to change our stride to accommodate walkies or suffer any harmful helpers. The two of us roll together at the pace of pride.

Walking, it turns out, is overrated. It's weird to me that walking is the obsession of many nondisabled people. Why would we want to walk, when we can soar? Walking feels like such a chore. We move about the world with a freedom and flow that walkies don't enjoy. Wheels are freedom. On this, we seem to agree, when it comes to a bus, a bike, a train, or a car. In all of these transportation modes, we sit down and use wheels to propel us forward. We recognize the freedom that wheels empower, except when it comes to wheelchairs.

Using a wheelchair means there is no slapping our feet on the pavement, no tripping, no trotting along. There is floating, rolling like a river around every corner, powered by community. Jesus walked on water, so why can't I float?[1]

There are many wonderful ways to move about the world. We are not in a race. We can go at our own pace. Rolling is not inherently better than walking, just like walking is not superior to gliding. That's the point, isn't it? We all move and groove in a variety of ways. We need to stop controlling and categorizing the way we all show up. We need to stop powering through life like we're above resting. We need to stop turning every offer of help into a showdown. Holding fast to this truth is important for me to affirm my own dignity. It is also one way I reinforce to

1. Many thanks to my wise friend Brenna Jones for this. It turns out it wasn't too campy for me.

myself and to the world that I am enough, just as I am. Our ways of existing and creating community are valuable and don't require nondisabled people's understanding. Perhaps I am so steadfast in trashing trashy helpers because it is one area where it feels clear that I have the power to affirm that I am enough and my "no" is enough.

Disability is not an invitation to trash or dismiss. Whether people realize it or not, we are living our own bliss. Much of what I think is happening in these moments with harmful helpers is that they are confronted with their own helplessness of not knowing how to be in community with us. Or, they are worried they will join us one day. We are the Ghost of Christmas Yet to Come, and to many, that's more frightening than the scourge of Scrooge.

Whatever the reason, harmful helpers display myths about disabled people that are tired and untrue. How embarrassing for them. Our knowledge, our experience, our very beings are valuable, even though we are so often trashed.

I wish people knew how treasured disabled people were, are, and will always be. Maybe then, we wouldn't have to carry this weight alone. I want to resist the narrative that extricates our worth—the one that says we need to be "valuable" members of society to be treated with dignity and respect. I want to resist only praising our contributions that can be commercialized. We are inherently valuable because we are divine. But I also want to share the ways that our disability community is, and has always been, contributing to our world. So many disability cultural artifacts build community and co-flourishing for everyone.

Nuance matters. One idea expressed two ways can change the whole vibe. Tired: I don't have any kids (banal, boring). Wired: My bloodline stops with me (mysterious, mythical). Same idea, different impact. We might say the same for the difference between a butt dial and a booty call. They have the same denotation but a very, very different connotation. I learned this the hard way when I mixed them up in class.

Nuance is important when we talk about our experiences as a disability community, because our stories are so often co-opted or commodified. When I say that we are valuable, I mean that nothing and no one can take away that we are divine. I also mean that our disability community's presence, wisdom, and creativity have benefited all of us. Disabled people know how to solve problems and facilitate community in ways nondisabled people haven't had to consider. Take everything from our community's innovations to our expertise in remote community-building. Disabled people practice the power of possibility-making. It is not just that we shouldn't be trashed, it is that we are already co-creating new ways of being together—in person and online—that allow all of us to thrive.

The moment we reach the sensory room, I notice a shift. Not a cataclysmic one at first, but it is definitely there, lingering in the edges of experience. Relaxed shoulders is where it starts. Shoulders no longer befriend the ears and settle into their own real estate down below. Jaws unclench. Then, brows unfurl. Deep exhales abound. Before I know it, I look around at the four students exploring the sensory room, and they are stretched out, on the floor, relaxing. At rest. At peace.

It's a rare occurrence for university students to be at ease. "There aren't many places on campus where I would feel comfortable enough to sit on the floor," a Black autistic student admitted to me later. She is someone who stands on business. To witness her share how she is at ease speaks volumes about the sanctity of space. Most other spaces ask her to mask her internal body signs.

In its essence, the sensory room is just like any other conference room on campus. A ten-foot-by-twelve-foot space, it could have been just another room, until I asked if we could make it a sensory space for our students.

Regardless of whether students identify as autistic, neurodivergent, or disabled, sensory rooms provide holistic benefits. In both quantitative and qualitative studies, sensory rooms soothe and smooth energy levels.[2] They also benefit overall mental health. Mood. When used in school settings, sensory rooms increase students' ability to become more engaged in class.[3] In other words, sensory rooms are a sensation. But they are not only for when you're overwhelmed or overstimulated. One study found that sensory rooms support emotional regulation and offer alternative stress management strategies.[4]

Life is busy, busy, busy. So ubiquitous is living life with back-to-back meetings and towering to-do lists that when a meeting ends even four minutes early, someone trumpets they are "giving you your time back." Wow, how generous. How will I spend my wild and precious four minutes? Let me count the ways.

Sadly, many of us know how much we can cram into just four minutes in our attention economy. Time to grab a snack pack, skip to the loo, and fill up a water bottle too. It's a lot. Nobody wins, but everybody loses. Forget sweet dreams. "I'll sleep when I'm dead" is more the vibe. We're micro-dozing.

The sensory room is one way to change the story we tell ourselves about ourselves, which is powerful and potent. If we tell ourselves that this is the way it has to be, we won't bother investing

2. Nastaran Doroud, Matthew Cappy, Kaleb Grant, Mason Scopelliti, Carol McKinstry, and Devlyn McMahon, "Sensory Rooms Within Mental Health Settings: A Systematic Scoping Review," *Occupational Therapy in Mental Health* 41, no. 1 (2025), https://doi.org/10.1080/0164212X.2024.2308290.

3. Emilie Brzack, Olivia DeWeerd, and Erica Roll, "Program Evaluation of the Impact of Sensory Room Interventions on Student Readiness in Muskegon County," thesis/dissertation, Grand Valley State University, July 2019, https://scholarworks.gvsu.edu/ot_pediatrics/15.

4. Stephanie Haig and Christopher Wagstaf, "A Mixed Methods Study into the Effectiveness of Sensory Rooms in Reducing Agitation Levels in a Psychiatric Intensive Care Unit," *Journal of Psychiatric Intensive Care* 20, no. 2 (September 2024): 67–77.

in rewriting the narrative when it doesn't work. We know that rush is rotting us. We know that the quick pace kicks us in the face. We know that lights, smells, and sounds resound louder for some than others, and that we can author a new chapter of community care together.

So I suggested we establish a sensory room for students, complete with therapeutic furniture, bubble walls, stim tools, and plenty of room to pace. It's needed to slow down in the rat race. The sensory room declares that we don't always need to be fighting and biting and plotting the course; we can chill and be still. Or we can wiggle and jiggle. There is not a singular "right" way to use a sensory room. The sensory room acknowledges that we all have access needs that deserve to be met, and that we get to be part of meeting access needs together as a community.

I think Jesus cares about meeting access needs. Jesus offers an access check-in when asking, "What do you want me to do for you?" (Mark 10:51). Jesus offers remote access to the centurion's servant (Luke 7:1–10).[5] Jesus speaks in plain language instead of the lofty language of the era. Surely Jesus recognizes the overstimulating chaos of crowds. He is always retreating to his own sensory-avoidant space by ditching the disciples to pray, grieve, and breathe. I think Jesus would enjoy our sensory room.

We have both sensory-seeking and sensory-avoidant spaces, recognizing that access needs fluctuate from day to day and hour to hour, and that what some find to be a refreshing space, others find radioactive. One person's calm is another person's chaotic. While the sensory room is curated from the wisdom of our neurodivergent community, everyone is welcome to participate, and that's exactly what has happened.

The biggest surprise of the sensory room hasn't been that students are using it. I knew that they would, even when there was

5. I am using "remote access" here as a term to express the way Jesus does not require the centurion's servant to travel to experience Jesus's presence. Instead, Jesus creates the conditions for access to community without physical presence.

skepticism before it was built. I knew they would because I have learned the disability wisdom that meeting access needs benefits all of us, regardless of how we identify or associate.

The biggest surprise has been how quickly something that was once revolutionary has become routine. Every time I pass the sensory room, I notice students and staff utilizing the space. It is one that is rejuvenating, and the students relish it. Who can blame them?

It's been delightful to witness how the sensory room has so quickly become a mundane manifestation of our students' access needs and how we can proactively meet them as a community. No longer does anyone question the existence of the sensory room, nor does anyone doubt its bountiful benefits. In a matter of months, the sensory room has gone from radical to regular.

The space meets our students' access needs, to be sure. But it also serves a critical cultural function in proclaiming that our access needs are worthy of being met without proving you are disabled "enough." It takes up space—literally—in an environment where space is often politicized and productivity is praised. It declares that rest is not just nice but necessary for each one of us. It proclaims that every member of our community is valuable. It acknowledges what we know to be true: that each of us is divine, just as we are, and that no one can take that from us.

The sensory room is a space where we get to experience the world we want to live in. That world is brimming with resting, stimming, and dimming lights. And it is sacred. The room is an active, living, ongoing invitation for the community to express our internal body signs and meet our access needs. The invitation doesn't expire. It gives students permission to explore their own disability experience and serves as a soft landing for their ongoing formation. Beanbags included. This practice stems from the small but mighty idea that the disability community is valuable and that our disability wisdom is a gift to the community.

In this way, we are discipling the next generation to treat their bodyminds as temples. We don't need to enshrine the shame and stigma of society, spreading negative messages about neurodivergence, when we get to be a part of creating a world where all are welcome as our full selves. Stigma strips people of their humanity. It turns a whole person into a singular quality. Reductive, much? It treats people like trash, even if you don't throw it at them. The sensory room restores what stigma has stripped away. It says, "We've been expecting you, and we are so glad you are here!" There is no need to cloak yourself in shame, because we want you here. Taste and see, the sensory room is good.

Disability justice activists Stacey Park Milbern and Leah Lakshmi Piepzna-Samarasinha describe disability identity experience as a type of rebirth. They state the importance of learning "how our bodyminds evolve in their crip, neurodivergent, Deaf, sick identities over time," and they emphasize that this is not a static identity but one that shifts as new strategies emerge.[6] They advocate for a paradigm shift from understanding disability as a type of death to acknowledging disability as a rebirth. We might call this becoming a new creation.

For disabled people, this process isn't just about learning about our own access needs or uncovering the pieces of ourselves we've learned to mask; it is also about unlearning the stigma that we have inherited about disability. It is an individual and communal process that allows us to learn how valuable disability truly is. The sensory room is just one place where disabled students get to unlearn some of the shame of stimming and instead give it a new name; a place where they are part of a community of care and get to thrive.

6. Stacey Park Milbern and Leah Lakshmi Piepzna-Samarasinha, "Crip Lineages, Crip Futures: A Conversation by Stacey Park Milbern and Leah Lakshmi Piepzna-Samarasinha," in *Crip Genealogies*, ed. Mel Y. Chen, Alison Kafer, Eunjung Kim, and Julie Avril Minich (Duke University Press, 2023), 104. They specifically talk about how important it is to do this work in community with queer BIPOC elders and leaders.

I want the sensory room to be the place to be. Not some stuffy space that requires you to perform your disability in one way that fits neatly within our expectations, but a community space that is made by and for our community. The sensory room has space to lounge, to pace, to breathe, to move. All the sensory tools are for students to groove. There are no disability doubters asking if you *really* need to use the room. It is a space where no one assumes, where no documentation is needed to prove you are disabled enough. No critique, just community, with no need to bluff. No need to identify in one particular way. We know access needs fluctuate from day to day. The sensory room is open to anyone to use, with toys and tools freely given for students to choose.

It's not just for disabled people. The sensory room benefits all of us. For me, the sensory room is just another example of how valuable disability wisdom is. It is the antidote to the limiting stories that began this chapter. Instead of trashing us, transform with us.

We are not developing an accessibility checklist but discipling a community on how to value access, disability wisdom, and care. The sensory room is a radical celebration of disability culture and the value it brings to our community. It's not just for us but for everyone.

PRACTICE

Color the world that we want to co-create. We know that coloring in, doodling, and drawing is good for us. As you consider the ways you are (un)learning, use this as a tool and technique. Make our world vibrant!

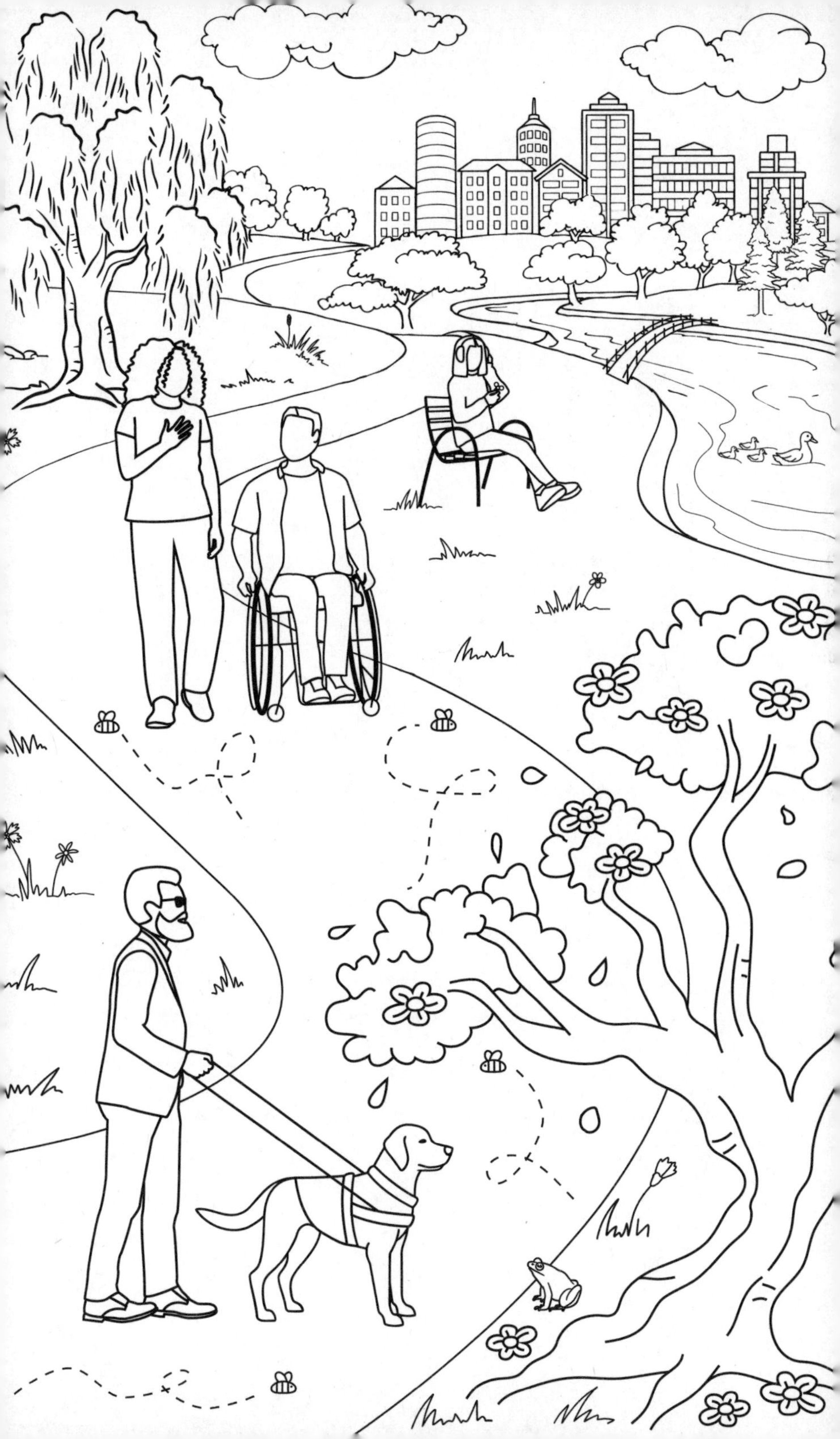

9

MY DISABILITY IS ADAPTABLE

Jesus is bad at math. With just a couple of fish and five loaves, Jesus and the community feed over five thousand people. Jesus knows there is enough, regardless of what the ROI recommends. Jubilee cancels debt so people don't have to work their assets off.[1] The liberation that abounds in Scripture cannot be found in a P&L. So it tracks that kin-dom living doesn't really make fiscal sense.[2] Just ask Zacchaeus.

When we meet him, he's "a chief tax collector and was rich" (Luke 19:2). He seems like someone who would Excel at spreadsheets. It's easy to bad-mouth Zacchaeus because he represents something most of us find tedious: paying taxes. (But why are there so many tax forms? 1040, 1099, I-9, W-2. They sound more like droids from *Star Wars* than tax chores. There's no accounting for it. It's so taxing.)

1. Check out Leviticus 25 for more on the year of Jubilee, which restored people's land, cancelled debts, released anyone who was enslaved, and provided rest for people and land alike.

2. For more on kin-dom, check out Ada María Isasi-Díaz, "Kin-dom of God: A Mujerista Proposal," in *In Our Own Voices: Latino/a Renditions of Theology*, ed. Benjamin Valentin (Orbis Books, 2010), 171–90.

Zacchaeus participates in a system that our society deems acceptable. Who cares if it is draining to those around him? That's not *his* problem. It's a rich man's world. He just wants to be audit he can be in accrual world. He didn't plot the system that oppressed his neighbors, nor is he responsible for it. Or so he thinks. After Jesus invites himself over, Zacchaeus proclaims, "Half of my possessions, Lord, I will give to the poor, and if I have defrauded anyone of anything, I will pay back four times as much" (Luke 19:8).

Zacchaeus doesn't waste time defending his doctrine. He doesn't absolve himself via an intent loophole or narci-gesis. He doesn't ask for the chapter and verse of where it says he should care about people. He doesn't blame the budget or cook the books. He directly acknowledges that he has the means to restore, and restores. That's it. That's the thesis.

And Jesus? It is worth noting that Jesus describes Zacchaeus's response as "salvation." According to Jesus, this defiant fiscal faithfulness is what saves Zacchaeus, not just his bottom line. Jesus calls Zacchaeus a "son of Abraham," affirming his inherent identity as divine (Luke 19:9). Zacchaeus uses the sycamore-fig tree as a type of accessible seating, finagling access on the fly, and Jesus meets him there with a rooted grace that bears fruit.

We have too often relegated the divine exclusively to the spiritual realm, as though our lives can be compartmentalized like trash and recycling bins. Paper and plastic to the left, all spiritual scraps to the right. But, as Zacchaeus shows us, kin-dom living impacts *all* aspects of our lives. There is no separation of sacred and secular. There is no "us" and "them." Bethany McKinney Fox even reads this story as a healing narrative for this disabled man because his life flourishes by giving his possessions away.[3] Healing

3. Bethany McKinney Fox, *Disability and the Way of Jesus* (InterVarsity, 2019), 144–45. For more on Zacchaeus and disability, check out Amos Yong, "Zacchaeus: Short and Un-Seen," *Christian Reflection: A Series in Faith and Ethics* (2012): 11–17, https://ifl.web.baylor.edu/sites/g/files/ecbvkj771/files/2022-12/Disability StudyGuides.pdf.

is not about physically changing but about transforming how we think about coin and community.

Jesus doesn't shame or blame Zacchaeus for his disability or try to alter it. Instead, he dines with Zacchaeus and defines righteousness by halting any hoarding mentality rooted in wealth and not in worth. This echoes Jubilee's emphasis on restoration by redistributing wealth. It also highlights how our disabled elder Zacchaeus was, is, and always will be divine.

It is my experience that church folks generally portray themselves as sinners: unworthy, lowly, even worm-like sinners. Until it comes to ableism (or its cousins, racism, queerphobia, and misogyny), where we assume that we are well-intentioned and give ourselves the benefit of the doubt because of the intent loophole. "I didn't mean it that way!" saves the day. This is not the way.

Zacchaeus isn't like that. He shows radical generosity, right here and now. He does not pass Go or collect $200. He does not seek a monopoly on extortion. His generosity is not driven by guilt or charity but is done out of sincerity. Zacchaeus gets real about his fiscal and social privileges. He repays four times what he took in a system that he didn't design, but he doesn't bother blaming the system or claiming that it doesn't make cents. "The way things are" doesn't balance the budget. Zacchaeus's radical generosity is a reparation for the community, a return to the co-flourishing of Jubilee.

We get to repair what is broken.

Reparation is about responding to injustice by paving the way for a more just future. Scripture emphasizes the work of repair and reconciliation: between us and God, us and one another, and us and the community of creation. We are called to breathe life into places that are considered too dead to invest in, like the laundromat and the park. We declare that the kin-dom of heaven is the one that we want to build, not any empire of materialism, consumerism, or self-preservation. Jesus math does not add up. Jubilee cannot be contained by capitalist accounting. We get the joy of participating in repairing, restoring, and reviving. Sometimes with our will and often with our wallets. Who *wouldn't* want to be a part of that?

We can follow the disability wisdom of Zacchaeus to focus on reparation. For some of us, this will include a change to finances, fourfold. For others, a shift in the ways we show up. For all of us, it will require that we are more invested in restoration than who is responsible or even who is right. Justice is more important than justifying ourselves. May we follow the example of our disabled elder by choosing reparation over rebuttal.

We have the power to repair what has been. This theology is not theoretical. I have had the privilege of witnessing people choose to change instead of estranging members of our community. Disability has a way of prompting the need to adapt, because society is built without us in mind. May these stories be a blessing and a call to action for us in how to adapt for the sake of co-flourishing.

"I want to share a story about my disabled son," a nondisabled parent interjects. My face winches together a smile, but my insides squirm, awaiting what kind of tall tale this will be. All too often, disabled people are props in someone else's story of service, objects instead of subjects, revealing how patient and pious someone is for *putting up* with us. But I want to give her a chance to surprise me, so I wait, willing for my wariness to be withdrawn.

She shares that her teen, a wheelchair user, didn't want her help wheeling through doors. (Can relate.) She ignored her son's petitions, dismissing them as too loud and proud. She wanted him to get a move on in every crowd. She wasn't focused on the fact that he could wheel himself about. She didn't want him left behind or left out. So she pushed him, despite his pleas and protests.

One day, she had an epiphany: Her need for speed wasn't helping at all. She *wanted* to support her son. Yet she realized "that was more about me than him." She was so focused on her son catching up with everyone else that she didn't realize she was rushing him for no reason. She was in a hurry and forced him to scurry. She'd fooled herself into believing this was for her son, but really, it was for her. She had to slow down and give her son space to go at his own pace. She had to learn to let go—literally—of her son's wheelchair.

When she's done telling her story, I am surprised by where it landed. Of course, no one can live independently, but she had to learn when to *not* intervene in her son's life just because he's disabled. Her chop chop needed to be given the chop. It is a micro-moment, but a meaningful one all the same. Something passes between us, like the aroma of a warm curry pie greeting you as you arrive home. May we always give people the chance to change.

I saw the sign. I almost didn't believe it at first. Whipping the car around, I did my best J-turn to give the sign a second read and believe it in my bones.

One gloomy Saturday afternoon, I drove past a Gothic Revival church with an orange vinyl banner out front proclaiming, "Celebrate accessibility! Our new ramp welcomes all through the same door." It is the first time I can ever remember a church *celebrating* accessibility. The year is 2025.

The 1923 fieldstone building was fashioned a generation before ADA, and yet this congregation constructed an accessible entrance so that all parishioners could enter through the front door. Not through a narrow alley with rodent droppings on the floor. Not through the back, where even getting there is a chore. I don't know the story of this particular ramp, but I wish for many more. I do know what the ramp's investiture signifies. It acknowledges that disabled people have been forced to enter our houses of worship through a different door, out the back, where only Mickey and Minnie reside.

I text a photo of the radiant ramp to my friend, who replies with a string of joyful emojis as both of us happy dance, our text chain aglow with the glory of access. I print a photo of the sign and pin it on the bulletin board in my office to remind myself of what's possible. Every person who comes by responds nearly the exact same way: "I've never seen a church do that before!"

One day, I hope that this response will no longer be true. I hope that this church's ramp will no longer be worthy of comment because access at church will have become so customary. I hope that our sanctuaries can provide sanctuary.

Somehow, I have hope that this will be the case. My hope is not the sugary stuff of wishes whispered over birthday cakes. It is the hope that we can draft a better world for all of us, not just those with bodyminds we currently call "nondisabled." Hope is the inner alarm inside your bones that tells you something is not right. Hope is the last dregs of gas in the tank after the burst of the fuel light. Hope is a flickering candle that the wind cannot deplete. I have a hard-won, rugged, "I get knocked down, but I get up again" hope that one day that statement will be obsolete. Not because I've been miraculously transfigured but because the world has been transformed.

The movie lights begin to fade. We are about to go somewhere we've never been before. Dazzling images on a huge silver screen. Sound that I can feel. The film is about to begin. The only problem? I am stuck in between a rocker seat and a hard place. Heartbreak doesn't feel good in a place like this.

I was excited to attend the premiere of a disability coming-of-age film, without the side of inspiration porn we have come to expect. *The Ride Ahead*, directed by disabled filmmaker Samuel Habib, tracks a rite of passage that many of us are familiar with: becoming an adult. According to Sam, "No one tells you how to be an adult, let alone an adult with a disability."

The show was sold out. The theater whirred with excited members of the disability community, friends, family, and allies, all delighted to cheer on one of our own. Disabled people rarely get a crack at telling our own stories. So when we do, the community shows up and shows out. Until, that is, the theater cracks under the pressure of us doing so.

Twenty-two wheelchair users showed up. This should be cause for celebration, but instead, it was cause for congestion. Or as we'd say in Australia, it was chockers. There were only six allocated spots for wheelchair users, which—go with me on this—is less than twenty-two. I'm no math major like Zacchaeus, but it doesn't add up.

The show must go on, I guess, because the lights faded and the credits rolled, even as many of us wheelchair users wondered, "What's the plan?" We watched while perched perpendicular to the screen. Many of us became fast friends because we were now sitting way too close to strangers for comfort. The theater was like an overstuffed suitcase. You know the type. You have to sit on it just to zip it up, and even then, the zipper is gasping, clenching, clinging to the fabric for dear life.

No wonder so many of us disabled people have so much emotional baggage. (Which I really think should be called "grief-case." What a missed opportunity.) Disabled people are used to the fact of our sheer existence surprising people. Even in a film that is by us and for us, the theater is not with us.

Our disability community is not expected to be out and about. People seem to think we're at home where we can pout. People expect that we'll be fewer or feebler and don't realize that we are already a vibrant part of the community. The film was so popular that too many people came to celebrate it. What a happy problem to have.

A happy problem, until their ignorance cooked up a fire hazard. We tripled the slated wheelchair user capacity, sardining ourselves into a space we simply did not fit but where we knew we belonged.

It was crammed, cramped, and chaotic. We are adept at adapting, finding access solutions on the fly, but the theater was a bottleneck. It was dehumanizing and deflating that even for a movie about disability, inaccessibility was the name of the game.

What's more, this theater had the amount of wheelchair-accessible seating that is legally required. This is just one reason why ADA is a floor and not a ceiling. The theater had enough ADA seating, but it still wasn't enough. ADA is not the metric of accessible. Instead, we need to design spaces and events so we can all flourish.

That's what I said in my email to the event organizers, anyway. I reached out to them to introduce myself and to share the demeaning experience with them in hopes of it becoming a learning opportunity. I reached out to them to offer to partner on designing a more accessible film festival.

What happened next was astonishing. The event organizers apologized. They made an actual apology acknowledging that the screening left "audience members feeling unsafe and dehumanized," alongside a commitment to do better in the future.

Next came a meeting. The organizers invited dialogue on how to improve. There were no cop-outs, fake-outs, or blow-offs. Typically, these "dialogues" feature more dodgers than a baseball game. Not here. They genuinely wanted to learn. They did the work. They hired an accessibility consultant. They wanted to do better.

And do better they did. The next year's festival featured movable seats to welcome as many wheelchair users as possible. There was a ramp to the stage for the panelists. "This was a really accessible venue!" exalted a guest who was unaware of the inaccessibility issues from the previous year. Accessibility became not just a pursuit but also a practice, so much so that it was felt and acknowledged by community members.

It took hard work, humility, and humanity. It required ego to not get in the way of equity. But it was worth it to build an accessible environment and experience. What sparkles to me about this experience isn't that the first screening was janky and jarring. I am used to that. What sparkles is that there was a willingness to learn beyond when people were watching. It is easy to performatively care about accessibility or to pretend, like a politician, that your mission has a tradition of contrition. Boy, bye. But there are very few people who are willing to do the work after the cameras stop rolling. There are very few who want to create access without shortcuts. There are very few who are willing to restore instead of rebut.

I hope we are some of the few.

Let's give people the space to surprise us. These stories might feel triumphant, but they all started in a place of tension. All of them are about mess-ups and muck-ups. All of them required transformation in order to make the community more accessible.

How it started: A mother pushed her teenager without consent or contemplation but a lot of rush. A church did not have a ramp for over one hundred years. A theater was ADA compliant but not accessible. People were crammed, slammed, and jammed at a film screening by us and for us. Such were some of you.

How it's going: People were more interested in mending than defending their actions.

One of the biggest barriers to creating a culture of access is ego—not from adversaries but from allies. It is a truth universally acknowledged that a disability ally in possession of a platform must be in want of strife. It is not just prejudice but pride that gets in the way of a culture of access. We start to think that we are not the problem, that we are not the ones creating inaccessible places or spaces. We start to think that it's those *other* Christians who are causing trouble.

The truth is that we will all mess up. We have a lifetime guaranteed of that. We will say the wrong thing. We will make an assumption that reveals how we've internalized stigma or stereotypes.

Most of us don't wake up in the morning hoping to be biased, yet bias still persists. The goal isn't to be perfect but pliable.

All of these stories started with ableism, whether intentional or not. But they didn't end that way. People were willing to do the work of creating a culture of access. In my experience, being willing to adapt is more important than being right. Being open to learning is more important than being knowledgeable. How we live our lives is more important to me than what we claim is our doctrine.

Something I notice about a lot of Christian communities is that we are more interested in proving the "other side" wrong than we are in making sure everyone can belong. Some of us have even left communities with harmful beliefs but haven't done the internal work of reexamining their corrupting corresponding practices. We are quick to cancel and slow to grow. I am not talking about staying in situations that are harmful to us. I am not recommending sucking it up or sticking it out. May our boundaries be blessed. Critique is a necessary tool to tell us what is wrong.

Yet criticism alone is not a community builder. Many of us ditch harmful beliefs only to pitch the exact same harmful practices. Canceling people because they get one word wrong, shutting someone out because they didn't meet our metric, shutting someone up who practices their faith in a different way than we do. We've decided which forms of direct action and mutual aid we value the most, and we've dismissed anyone who doesn't fit our mold. All of that feels satisfying in the moment (believe me, I know), but it doesn't give us the opportunity to learn and grow. Change typically requires a deeper commitment to community than casting out does. Zacchaeus is willing to pay four times as much because of how Jesus math multiplies. Jubilee is more about grace than holding a grudge.

Creator is constantly adapting for us humans. Whether it's through clothing, quail, kings, covenants, or companions, Creator meets humans where we are and accommodates us. From providing brothers to trees that "mother," Creator shows us how access is divine.[4] Adapting is hallowed work. I hope I am someone who gives people the chance to change and calls them into a more inclusive way. I hope I am someone who cares more about inviting people in than shutting people out.

The people whose stories fill this book are not evil, and I really believe they were not out to get me. In fact, I believe they have inherent worth and dignity. All of them are divine. Most of us are doing our best. Sometimes, our best still hurts the people around us. In these moments, it isn't all that helpful to lecture one another about the ideologies we thought we were upholding; it is more important to be willing to listen and learn for the sake of love. The moment we think we've got this whole Jesus thing figured out better than everyone else is the moment we can be certain we do not. I believe that we are capable of change.

The examples in this chapter are somewhat replicable. But more than that, I hope we take these stories and make them applicable to wherever we find ourselves. Our temperament in responding to being called in is more important than a how-to template. Community requires creativity, care, and change. Change doesn't have to be grand; it can be granular. We get to act elastic with one another and stretch for each other, instead of snapping. We get to build a community where accountability is more rampant than accusations, where growing is more valued than gossiping, where we acknowledge that we are all learning—not as an excuse but as an invitation. We get to be flexible so all can flourish.

May others also offer the same grace to us.

4. I am referring to Aaron, who is a divine accommodation to Moses, the sycamore-fig tree for Zacchaeus, and mother trees (mentioned in chapter 3).

PRACTICE

We have the power to change. Sometimes this can feel too macro, so let's make it micro together.

Option 1: Choose a word to cycle out of commission this week. Maybe the word is rooted in ableist nonsense. Maybe the word isn't honoring the divinity in each one of us. Come up with a replacement word to use instead. Whenever you find yourself about to say the chosen word, reach for the new one. Words can shape worldviews. The more we practice saying that we are divine, the more we will believe it.

Option 2: Choose a new habit to create a culture of access. Maybe it's turning on the captions during a Zoom meeting. Maybe it's putting alt text on your social media. Maybe it's getting noise-canceling headphones or sensory tools for your community. Whatever it is, make it doable without being daunting. Start small. We change by making new practices a part of our habits, day by day.

Changing our habits does not have to come with a side of shame. None of us are perfect, but all of us can become pliable.

10

MY DISABILITY IS RADIANT

The first time I used mobility aid superpowers, I was eleven. I wanted to turn off a light in the living room but didn't want to get up, so I used my crutches as a robotic arm to flick the light switch off. My brother and I chuckled. We wondered what else I could use mobility aids for.

Before long, I discovered that if you unfolded my collapsible cane in just the right way, it could land on its feet. Like flip cup, but for canes.

Next was transforming my high school mobility scooter into the Batmobile so I could become "The Cripped Crusader." My friend painted detachable cardboard wings that didn't get in the way of the wheels. Why didn't we make Wonder Woman's invisible jet, you ask? I ask myself the same question. Grace covers a multitude of sins.

At that time, Philippians 4:8 was scribbled on a scrap of paper on the lower right corner of our TV at home: "Whatever is true, whatever is noble, whatever is right, whatever is pure, whatever is lovely, whatever is admirable—if anything is excellent or praiseworthy—think about such things" (NIV). This was the era where TV was time-bound, where you stayed home on Sunday nights and yelled "It's on!" as soon as the TV blared, "My name is Sydney Bristow. Seven years ago, I was recruited by a secret branch of the CIA called SD-6 . . ." This was the era where you negotiated with your sister who got to go to the bathroom during which commercial break so you didn't miss a moment of Sydney working for the very people she thought she was fighting against.

I think my parents wanted us teens to think about that verse whenever we watched TV, played a board game, or hung out with friends. It was broadcast in the living room as a call (or maybe a caution). Despite my best espionage efforts, I was no double agent on *Alias*, but I did start to uncover the magnificence of mobility aids during this time. I am not sure my parents anticipated that, but the Philippians-clad living room was the backdrop for this all the same. Since then, I have grown up from requiring a specific chapter and verse to believe that something is true, right, or lovely, but I do think the values of that verse have been planted within my spirit all the same. I didn't know it then, but I was starting to experience the radiance of disability. I just didn't have the language for it yet.

I am using the word "radiant" as a powerful resistance to the ugly laws that once legally locked away disabled people from mainstream society and still echo in assumptions about whose bodyminds belong in public. I am using the word "radiant" to illustrate that disability is pure, lovely, admirable, excellent, and praiseworthy, and I want us to think about disability as such things. Disabled people are so often airbrushed or ambushed out. Describing disability as radiant is not about reproducing unrealistic beauty ideals that promote white supremacy, ableism, and fatphobia but about reclaiming our radiance as our own. Beauty can feel like a members-only club, with everyone striving for an unattainable ideal while judging each other for not reaching it. This kind of beauty is not something I am chasing or commending.

Historically, we haven't been valued, but make no mistake: Disability is radiant.

Look no further than AI-generated images to know this is true. Have you ever noticed how polished AI images are? They're creepy and they're kooky, mysterious and spooky, they're all together ooky, the AI family. There's something too doctored or dressed up about them all, as if they are devoid of the depth of details of humanity. They are just a bit *off*. Perhaps because they are not human.

Give us texture, give us moles; erasing our face's traces of living should not be the goal. Let us droop, let us sag, may our crow's feet and laugh lines give us the right to brag. We want stretchmarks, we want thick thighs, let's stop shaming the circles under our eyes. It's the lines of wrinkles mapped on our faces that make up the poetry of our stories. We're not clones that anyone can copy-paste. We are not AI slop, made in haste. It's our diversity of features that is delightful. Humans are more radiant than AI, not in spite of but because we are mere mortals. Every freckle is fabulous, every wrinkle is wisdom, every shadow is sacred.

Lately, I find myself wondering if the ick factor of AI-generated images can help us appreciate the radiance of disability. When we get weirded out by waxy caricatures, perhaps we can begin to marvel at the variety of features of our bodyminds. Folks who are blind, Deaf, or neurodivergent; people with IDD, psychiatric disabilities, or limb difference; anyone with a physical or sensory disability. We are all radiant. It's the rhythm of our spasms that is sublime. Our short statures and our creaky joints, our mugs, moves, and motions are what *make* us radiant. Maybe AI can generate a cultural shift in how we think about radiance, not as airbrushed but as authentic.

My painted cardboard Batmobile wheels are no more, but the flare remains. What began with teenage joy at the glow and glitter of our cultural artifacts has moved into how I understand our community. We don't need a bat signal to answer the call. We celebrate each other's disability gains, canes, and hacks. Or the way Harriet McBryde Johnson puts it, "We enjoy pleasures other people enjoy, and pleasures peculiarly our own. We have something the world needs."[1]

We *ooh* and *ahh* at the lights on someone's new wheels, thrilled that they can avoid smushing dog poop on the path. We dance around the kitchen. A dance without a name but choreographed to the hustle and flow of our bodyminds. One wheel a little to the left, a rotated chair, and plenty of laughter are the only lyrics we need. We don't shrink our bodyminds to take up less space. We expand our wheelspans to the flow of our kitchen choreography. We can turn a dance floor into a runway.

We celebrate someone's new cane with a sturdier base. This cane can stand on its own, which we know is a boon in the bathroom. We cheer someone on with neurodivergent-friendly *woo*s, understanding how even praise can prickle when it's overstimulating. We congratulate a new Deaf parent whose child "failed" the hearing test, and all they do is win.[2] Everybody's hands go up, and they stay there.[3]

Relationships are where it happens. It can't be replicated or commodified. Our disabled joy blossoms and blooms with each seed of our disability wisdom. It is not for anyone but us. Our joy comes from a life lived looking in, developing the expertise of being able to create—often out of chaos—on the fly. It is divine.

Disability is a site and source of radiance. Disability knowledge, expertise, and techniques give birth to innovative ideas. We are not just dazzling when we fit in or shrink down. With every hand flap and ASL clap, with every delay and sway, we shine. With our

1. Harriet McBryde Johnson, "Unspeakable Conversations," *New York Times*, February 16, 2003, https://www.nytimes.com/2003/02/16/magazine/unspeakable-conversations.html.

2. Of course, many d/Deaf people do consider themselves to be disabled. For more, check out Danny Ko, "D/deafness," in *Skin, Tooth, and Bone: The Basis of Our Movement Is Our People; A Disability Justice Primer*, 2nd ed. (Sins Invalid, 2019), 88–93.

3. Raising hands in the air while twisting and waving them is "applause" in ASL.

canes, chewies, crutches, CART, and community, we glow just as we are. We are golden.

"I don't need to see the ground to know I'm jumping," she belts out, playing the piano while wearing gold-studded platforms. She towers over the room, and not just because of the five-inch heels.

I remember the first time I heard my friend, recording artist, and cultural changemaker Lachi sing "Diseducation," a song she wrote about navigating everyone else's ableism as a Black, blind woman. The whole room was mesmerized by her. Lachi, whose name rhymes with Versace, turns the tables on anyone who says disability is deficient and proclaims *they* need a diseducation. She shifts the need for change back on nondisabled people, where it belongs.

Lachi exudes glamour and guts. Her music is magic. She fuses pop, dance, dub, trap, and electro house. Think Lauryn Hill meets Alicia Keys meets Doechii. She is opinionated, witty, and authentic, and invites us to be the same.

Whenever Lachi sings, she gives everyone permission to be unapologetically the fullest version of themselves. She celebrates outcasts, misfits, and anyone who is misunderstood ("the least of these" in spiritual speak). She doesn't do this by explaining or erasing the qualities that people so often cast aside. She does this by showcasing how radiant disability is.

She turns a visual description into a song. She explains to the audience how scatting comes from her neurodivergent experience. She thanks her disabilities in her sets. She's a professional!

Lachi sparkles. Literally. The studs on her shoes, the sequins on her dress, the rhinestones on her Glam Canes, the glitter on her nails, and her electric personality all shine. But what makes Lachi truly sparkle aren't her platforms—it's the way she uses her platform to build community and celebrate the radiance of her craft and that of other disabled artists. This isn't out of charity or box-ticking. This is shining a light on talent, talent the world has often dismissed because we are disabled. This is shining a light on how disabled people are divine.

Disability is radiant, if only the world would notice our shine.

If someone has been around disability culture for any amount of time, they likely know about Kinetic Light, an innovative disability arts ensemble that uses movement, light, and sound as part of their intersectional approach to performance. They are iconic.

Why? They built a customized multi-level ramp with slopes, peaks, and valleys as part of their piece "DESCENT," where the ramp becomes more than a set piece, a partner in the dance choreography. The piece invites us to reimagine power, sensuality, and disability through curves and swerves.

Another piece, "Wired," includes them flying through the air in their wheelchairs. Barbed wire is used as a way to think about disability, race, gender, and control. It is powerful, provocative, and exquisite. They defy gravity.

Sure, they fly. They blend technology, design, and dance to invite us to think about access, disability, race, queerness, and gender. They don't play by the rules of someone else's game. They ask us to rethink the limits of categories we've often taken for granted and to enter a different world altogether.

Seventh grade science class would have been a lot more interesting if Kinetic Light, instead of some stuffy old textbook, had taught us about kinetic energy. Sorry, Newton. The way they swerve, swivel, and spin is a lesson in how bodies in motion stay in motion. They won't be grounded by other people's notions of what their bodyminds can do.

They are innovators. Access isn't *just* a checklist, a core value, or a practice in their world. It is an invitation to create. Access is a site of possibility-making. It is an aesthetic that opens up possibilities for transformation. Access is an art. Kinetic Light developed haptic technology, spatialized audio description, and multi-sensory, immersive, embodied installations. They expand access as a way to demonstrate how to innovate and immerse audiences in a world where more is possible than what we have been told. They are the future.

One of the most sacred experiences I've ever had is getting to work with founder and artistic director Alice Sheppard; founding member, choreographic collaborator, and dancer Laurel Lawson; research fellow in technology and access Colin Clark; and dancer Tatiana Cholewa. Our friendship was forged in fire and is sustained by joy. They are brilliant and bold, but that's not what makes working with them sacred. It's sacred because they do not shrink or shirk, they shine.

Their art is intense yet intimate, immersive yet intellectual, and timely yet timeless. They move in a way that makes it clear that disability is a source of radiant, abundant creativity. While anyone can admire and appreciate their art, Kinetic Light is by and for disabled people. They are not merely proving a point about how disabled artists are artists. They can fly circles around other artists because they are in a league of their own.

Getting to experience the captivating energy that is a Kinetic Light performance is transformative, because they are confidently creating artifacts of disability culture that celebrate our inherent radiance. They move with all the fluidity of water and all the brazenness of fire.

Disability is radiant, if only the world would notice our shine.

The first thing I notice are two inflatable arms that would feel more at home at a car wash than at an art gallery. Their bright cherry tint bursts into an otherwise pale room. They reach across the room to one another, one puffs up as the other collapses. One points at a crinkly, creamy rock. The other outstretches its nylon palm and wiggles and jiggles—a common practice in the Deaf community when trying to get someone's attention. Powered by an air blower, the arms twist and shout, suspended in air and time, continuously repeating the same motion.

I'm sitting in front of *Attention*, a sculpture by Christine Sun Kim and Thomas Mader that is housed at the Whitney Museum in New York. The sculpture goes on forever. That is to say, the nylon arms are repeatedly vying for our attention. It's as if the Deaf community has been asking us hearing folks to pay attention to Deaf culture forever and ever. As if repeatedly asking for attention will erode the rock over time. The sculpture, like many of Kim's pieces in this exhibit, blends literal, conceptual, and emotional meanings to invite us into her world, often using ASL and Deaf culture as a starting point of connection.

The exhibit includes infographics that blast the gaps between Deaf and hearing worlds. One shows how she would sign common phrases. My favorite is "sorry not sorry," which in ASL becomes "sorry zero." There are the symbols of sound to show exclusion, inclusion, and isolation. Her charcoal sketches are filled with letters in all caps, fluttering around the room. Smudges scatter across the charcoals, as though the slippage between ASL and English smears the true meaning. English can't quite reach to fill the space that ASL enlivens.

In some of her pieces, Kim thickens the visual grammar of ASL to develop a sense of emotion or reverberation or to show how sound is a social currency, like when the camera cut off her ASL interpretation of the national anthem at the Super Bowl. She left it all on the field, because that's where they cut it. It reminds me of how Sara Nović says Deaf people have a greater spatial awareness than hearing people since ASL is a 3D language. Being immersed in Christine Sun Kim's art makes that very clear. You only have to watch her sign "rocket's red glare" to know how limited English is by comparison. Her work is visceral, vibrant, and vivacious.

My favorite of her works is her series on Deaf rage. Who knew a bunch of charcoal pie charts could evoke such gut-wrenching anger? In it, Kim shares her experiences of Deaf rage through corresponding pie charts and angles. Deaf rage at someone leaving her suitcase on the tarmac because the flight attendant yelled out whose it was. No interpreters in meetings. Splitting artist's commissions with 'terps. Years of dealing with friends or family who don't bother to (learn) sign. Someone who offered her a wheelchair or a braille menu at restaurants after learning she's Deaf. As though all disabled people are the same. As though all access needs are alike. People being scared of us. People acting like we don't exist. Hell hath no fury like a woman scorned, and society has scorned her over and over again.

Hilarious and scathing, Christine Sun Kim's work gives us permission to rage. To rant. To rave at the world's ableist nonsense. Her art is accessible in form and content, inviting people to experience a world that they might never have conceptualized. Her righteous fury is unfurled on the page and sculptural stage for all to witness. She is not afraid to name and shame the toxic behaviors that she endures. #SorryZero.

Her art is radiant, if only the world would notice its shine.

"I didn't know I could like poetry," a student confesses. We're in a workshop where Douglas Kearney, a poet, professor, and librettist, shared how his creative process emerged from his processing style. He was taking notes on poetry one day when he realized that the way he processes information and takes notes *is* the poem. What if a poem didn't have to be linear? What if a poem could express everything, everywhere, all at once?

Insert neurodivergent poetics, a type of performative typography he designed.[4] Picture a Wordle-style collage that plays with

4. Douglas Kearney, *I Imagine I Been Science Fiction Always* (Wave Books, 2025).

font size, style, and structure. *That's* the poetry—less Shakespeare blank verse and more *Into the Spider-Verse*. Pow! Wham! Bam! It's less ABAB and more zip, zing, kroom, BOOM!

There is no beginning and no end. The reader can start in any place in the poem and read the words in any order. It's not just about the text but the texture. The reader's own order, cadence, and breath co-creates what the poetry can be each time the poem is read. The poems are new every morning. Great is thy poetry!

Neurodivergent poetics is Kearney's way of exploring the simultaneity and multiplicity of stimming. Instead of trying to use the form of the poem to contain or constrain his stimming, Kearney allows stimming to be a generative portal of creativity.

The result? His poetry packs a punch. Neurodivergent folks are often told, "You're doing too much. You need too much. You *are* too much." Or that stimming is distracting at best and dangerous at worst. People are told to mask their internal body signs in both explicit and implicit ways. Instead of falling in line, Kearney disrupts the whole idea that order and linear structure are necessary for meaning-making. Instead of masking, Kearney makes space for more Black neurodivergent folks to share their internal worlds through poetry.

Drawing from jazz, ragtime, and hip-hop, he invites us on a journey of playful disorientation in his poems. His poetry invites us to play. We get to be a part of the call-and-response journey of his poems because of the creativity generated by his neurodivergent experience. There's a musicality of movement in disregarding the structure so often imposed. Access needs are not a constraint but a creative tool in his neurodivergent poetics.

Disability is radiant, if only the world would notice our shine.

"Is there even such a thing as disability culture?"

I am asked this at least once a week. It's wild to me that people ask this question about such a large and vibrant community.

Imagine if we could reshape what we have been taught about disability to consider the artistry of our community. I wish people could know that we are radiant and notice our shine.

It seems that when disability and art are mentioned in the same sentence, it's usually about art therapy. Art is good for disabled people, we're told. But disabled people are also good for art.

It was this premise that led me to curate annual student art showcases. *ACDC: Art Celebrating Disability Culture* features art in different mediums sharing disability experiences from our students' perspectives.

One year, a student wrote and performed a poem entitled "Dear Future Blind Girl," dedicated to her younger self. "Blindness, I've discovered, is a way of living," she declares in her poem, which features the scents and soundscape that she draws upon to navigate the world. The smell of popcorn, the clank of metal, and the texture of velvet all become poetry that—according to her—she wouldn't otherwise connect to. Her blindness is not only her way of living but also her art form in crafting poetry.

Another student coded an animation of a boxy cartoon, dancing to shifting seasons in the background. Think *Bluey* meets *Minecraft*. For as long as this student could remember, people would ask him, "Why are you moving around so much?" The animation answers that question, syncing movement to his internal body signs, inviting the audience to experience his inner world. The movement of his Black body is no longer seen as a danger, a disruption, or a distraction but as an invitation to dance to the rhythm of the animation. In coding the piece, the artist shares a vibrant experience of neurodivergence where we can understand his internal body signs as a moving, grooving art form. Or the way he tells it, the animation prompts us to ask, "Why not move *more*?!"

Another artist used spoons as a painting practice. Instead of pushing past the pain when low on spoons, or masking her chronic pain, she allowed her bodymind to determine the pace of painting. This led to a layered effect in the painting, creating a unique style that otherwise would not have emerged without disability wisdom.

Our students use disability as a catalyst for creativity in both form and content. They display the radiance of our community—not in spite of but *because of* our diverse disabilities. They show us how lovely, admirable, excellent, and praiseworthy disability (art) can be by divulging the depths of their experiences. They don't shy away from naming the pain or politics of disability either. It is the authenticity of their experiences that is radiant.

Another student painted bright, abstract orange and yellow hues with broad tools to support manual dexterity. It's as if Kandinsky met Rothko in a petri dish. Thick strokes caked on the canvas as a result, giving the painting heft and gravitas. Disability as form forges possibilities for art to expand.

Ballet Folklórico Mexicano de Georgetown featured one student wearing a white lace Veracruz dress and the other wearing all black. These students wanted to capture the disability wisdom of interdependence, so they choreographed "El Cascabel" so that one dancer displayed brisk *zapateado* (the footwork) while the other dancer performed flowing *faldeo* (the skirtwork). Their dance displayed the interdependence of graceful and high-speed moves in a captivating, choreographed way. The two dancers never touched but were deeply intertwined in interdependence. Afterward, a colleague noted to me how much they thought the piece was like perichoresis, or the Trinity dancing together, which is the type of reference that really slaps at a Jesuit university.

Another student shared an ode to their crutch. One group celebrated Deaf culture through Bhangra. Another painted their experience of hallucinations. One student's photography explored what it means to leave a trace in a world that often overlooks what it cannot explain. One student painted a watercolor series featuring a woman wearing an orange hanbok in a shadowy bamboo forest to retell Korean mythology foregrounding disability. A walker and wheelchair user disrupted our expectations of dance through stillness, pausing with the power of communal breath to craft calmness. Alt text as poetry. Textured tapestry celebrating disability joy. Stamps to celebrate the perception of imperfection and the inherent politics of disability identity. Neurodivergent poetics. And the list goes on.

ACDC features artists who identify as blind, Mad, Deaf, Hard of Hearing, and spoonies, as well as people with IDD, apparent and nonapparent disabilities, and those with a complex relationship to the disability community and the term "disabled." There is no right way to be disabled and no terminology we enforce. Crip cards are not the cost of admission. We know you don't need to identify as disabled to experience disability or ableism. At ACDC, some students sit on the stage, some stand, some prerecord a presentation, some write a blurb for the emcee to share, and some don't come onstage at all. Some students show up with their pieces half done, but they fully show up. There is no pressure of performing participation. ACDC is a messy masterpiece, emphasis on messy.

The real radiance of ACDC isn't so much the dazzling art pieces or the skill level of our amazing students but the community cultivated in the presence of creativity. It's the way disability wisdom is on display from many who have never been considered theologians or teachers.[5] Most students haven't given themselves permission to create, and many have been taught that the product is more important than the process. But creativity is a value in and of itself. Creativity is true, right, pure, lovely, admirable, excellent, and praiseworthy. It is not the product but the process of creativity that is radiant. Disability is distinctive in its glow. No, I don't mean our pretty personalities, proclaimed with all the shade of Aretha Franklin purporting that Taylor Swift has "beautiful gowns." I

5. For more on how the world's greatest theologians are those who aren't considered theologians, in a different context, check out Kat Armas, *Abuelita Faith: What Women on the Margins Teach Us About Wisdom, Persistence, and Strength* (Brazos, 2021), 19–38.

mean we shine, shimmer, and sparkle. Disability is a creative force that has been instilled in us. Every time we create, we share our inner world with one another in hopes of co-creating a new one where all bodyminds are relished as radiant. We radiate the divine to the rest of the world, whether folks realize it or not.

Art is not just good for us—we, disabled people, are good for art.

PRACTICE

Take a psalm, poem, or song and create your own word collage. There is no wrong way to do this, but here are some ideas you might want to play with:

- What words do you want to make big?
- What words or images do you want to make bold?
- What icons, symbols, or graphics do you want to use? Think comic book, collage, and word art.
- What can be placed at an angle or in a corner?
- How can you play with the form to resist the norm?

Here is an example:

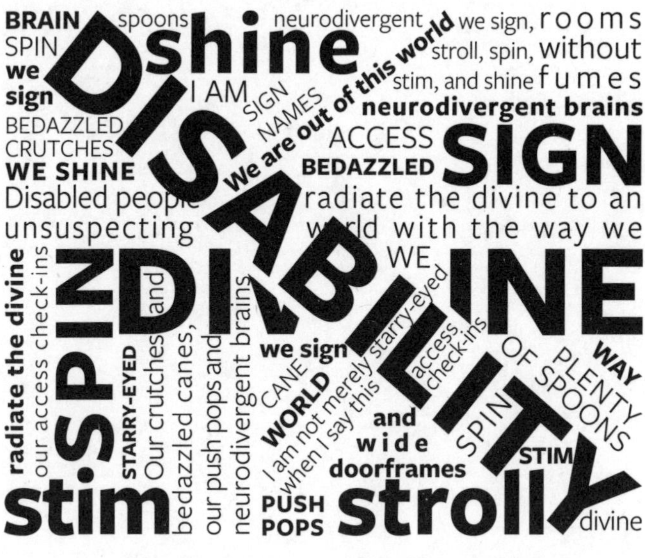

Once you have made your word art, reflect on how this allowed you to connect with the meaning. What did this hone or highlight for you? How did this practice breathe life into the piece?

11

MY DISABILITY IS JOYFUL

The second time her suitcase strikes my wheelchair, she calls me a C-you-next-Tuesday. I am in her way, she spits out. After I ask this stranger—who is flanking me with her suitcase in a thirty-second elevator ride—not to hit me again, she replies that she "didn't know." What, I am not sure. Perhaps she meant she didn't know she couldn't ram her suitcase into me. She didn't know she couldn't walk all over me. She didn't know these wheels don't negate the fact that I am human. It's no use. She continues the abuse and rams me again. Stranger: strike three. It's not until my husband asks her not to hit me that she skulks. The word of a nondisabled man is always heeded more than a disabled woman's.

I leave the elevator with the threads of my dignity frayed but knitted together by my resolve. I can't yarn on the elevator raider for long because I am met with a new aggressor, this one more nature than nurture: ice, ice, baby. I try not to slip on the icy ooze, but it has me stop, levitate, and listen. Ice is back to grab my attention. I can't wheel myself in my manual wheelchair (Rolland) when no one bothers to salt or snowplow, so I ask my spouse to steer me. I don't *want* to go speed skating, but that doesn't stop my wheelchair from drifting, lifting several centimeters in the air.

Before we know it, we are spinning the pavement on our very own ice-skating rink. Our double axel isn't particularly nimble, but it is quick; we manage to narrowly avoid a child making snow angels and a delivery Bike Angel whooshing past. By the time we stop gliding, there's nothing to do but laugh. The next time we slip and slide (on the very next block), we are grinning with all the joy of a dog mid-zoomie. Chuckling gives way to cackling in no time. Even our shoulders join in. Tears of glee leap from my eyes.

We land a 360 at 5th and Olive, courtesy of the slippery slush now masquerading as a sidewalk. We're doing our best Michelle Kwan or Kristi Yamaguchi, in my mind at least. In reality, it is more topsy-turvy, shake-and-bake-y. My wheelchair is now an unpredictable merry-go-round that spins us right round, baby, right round. Would recommend. Walkies are missing out.

People glare at us with more confusion than curiosity. It's not just the elevator raider. At one point, a woman leers at us for so long that I whisper "boo" to her. She scurries away before I can ask what she was gaping at. We are here for gawks and giggles. I used to hope they were admiring my wheels—bright, colorful, vibrant art. Rolland's spoke guards are adorned with a pair of Izzy wheels that twirl waves of electric purple, cobalt, and canary with each revolution. But on the slushy sidewalk, too many people stare at me for too long for me to convince myself of this fib. They are looking at me—at my torso, my thighs, my disabled body. They are looking at us, a nondisabled man and a disabled woman laughing too loudly for what people have come to expect from a wheelchair user. Evidently, we are supposed to be teary, weary, and dreary.

This is what it's like being in an inter-abled relationship. Eyes crawling all over my body, searching for answers to questions we are not asking. Why are you together? How does this relationship work? Won't he get tired of "taking care of" you? People project their own fear of disability onto us, as though we are a freak show they can ogle at. Step right up, come one, come all—there's a disabled woman who is joyful after all. How could it be? Come and see! Marvel at her, if you please. It's as though we need their permission to be in love.

"You're so lucky to have someone who will *put up with* your disability," a woman in front of us in line for mochas informs me. Translation: I can't expect much from life. Disabled people are treated as burdens everywhere we go.[1] We are silenced while our loved ones are given the mic. We are the target of relational violence that is too often cast as mercy because people cannot develop an imagination for our lives outside of burden ballads and pity parties. Limiting ideas about disability have real-world consequences for us.

People expect that disabled people will be more grim than grin. Nothing could be further from the truth. My disabled life is joyful, not in spite of but often because of my disability. Yes, being disabled in a world not built for my bodymind can be grating, berating, and frustrating. Being in pain is no picnic. Yet there is also levity and laughter. Disability is complex and complicated and contains a wide range of human emotions, joy prominent among them.

When people realize that we are a couple, they take it upon themselves to remind me how lucky I am. "What a relief you took vows to stay with one another in sickness and in health," cloaking their fear in platitudes, as though our marriage is a spouse trap, an obligation to shame him into staying with me. It's a trap!

My disability isn't a punishment or penance for my spouse. Sure, it comes with all kinds of unwanted stares, glares, and advice masked as care, but my disability is not his cross to bear. My

1. Kwame Anthony Appiah, "Is It OK to Dump Him Because of His Medical Condition?," *New York Times*, June 9, 2020, https://www.nytimes.com/2020/06/09/magazine/is-it-ok-to-dump-him-because-of-his-medical-condition.html.

disability isn't a test or a trap or a trial. I am human, and my needs are human.

Some of the irony is that my wheels are what stabilized Andrew so he didn't faceplant on the slushy calling itself a sidewalk. Without Rolland's handlebars, Andrew would be belly up on the boulevard. My wheels are what supported both of us, enough to make this street-side Slip 'N Slide more slide than slip. My wheels are what turned ice, ice, baby from vice to nice.

There's an intimacy that is forged by interdependence, of helping someone put on their socks frequently enough to know how much wiggle room they want for their toes. Or letting someone use the storage in your mobility scooter as a satchel. Our relationship thrives on the intimacy and joy that interdependency brings. We don't have a bad romance; we just want to dance on every snowcapped sidewalk. Let them cast us as villains and vixens. We know the truth: There are no burdens or saints in our relationship. Just love.

We know most people don't get our inter-abled love story. But we are too busy soaring to care, roaring with laughter as we're gone in a wink, making every sidewalk our ice-skating rink.

Everyone stares at us, but we don't care. We rush down the sloped sidewalk too quickly to respond to their abled gaze, to their wondering a little too loudly whether it's "safe for a wheelchair" to go *that* fast. The wind caresses our faces as we glide downhill, my wheels gaining momentum the faster we roll. We swoosh past their sneers, their fears, their leers at an inter-abled couple's joy. They flash past us so quickly, we are whizzing too fast to dwell. Wheels hover above the ground and we are flying—arms, wheels, and joy propelling us, laughter the only soundtrack we leave in our wake.[2]

2. Some of this appeared in Amy Kenny, "Love Stories: No Burdens or Saints, Just Love," Shondaland, February 25, 2022, https://web.archive.org/web/20230201225621/https://www.shondaland.com/live/family/a39211620/love-stories-no-burdens-or-saints-just-love.

There are plenty of funny stories in Scripture, and ample amounts of joy. Elijah loves toilet humor (1 Kings 18:27). Samson hulks out and takes the city gates as a souvenir (Judg. 16:3). There's that time Paul drones on for so long that someone falls asleep, falls out the window, and kicks the bucket (Acts 20:7–12). Sometimes I think we're out of practice at making space for joy. Why so serious? Many of us seem to be taught that spirituality is serious and therefore must be stale. I think Jesus would love a good "hill to die on" joke. Nailed it!

In my experience, disabled people know how to make space for the complexity of joy. When I am with disabled friends, I can relax because I am no longer the object of scrutiny, stares, and unsolicited advice. I can rest in the blessed assurance that my access needs will not be a shock or mocked. Even when access needs cannot be met, there will be a mutual understanding that they are valid. I can make sarcastic jokes about my own bodymind without people shrieking in horror. Our joy is based on the knowing laughter of people who get it.

When I am with people who get it, we make space for the variety of ways we come to, learn about, and experience our disabilities, knowing that there is not one "right" way to be disabled. We recognize that our other identities impact our experience of disability too. We know that when we have fun, people will use and abuse us for inspiration porn, and yet we choose to have fun anyway.[3] We know that we cannot do it alone. We name our limits and embrace interdependent support. We honor the power of disability joy. We develop networks of community care.

Of course, any place there are humans, there are human problems. Our disability community is no different. There are debates and disagreements about how to deal with accountability

3. Maysoon Zayid and Stella Young came up with the term "inspiration porn." Check out Stella Young, "Inspiration Porn and the Objectification of Disability," posted May 13, 2014, by TEDx Talks, YouTube, 9 min., 26 sec., https://youtu.be/SxrS7-I_sMQ.

and power. There is access friction. There are complicated ways that people are still unlearning what it means to *not* be the only disabled person in a room. There are ways that interdependence doesn't always occur no matter how badly you want it. Racism and lateral ableism run rampant. I do not wish to portray the disability community in a sugary, simplistic way, because we are human and we have chaos and cuts among the camaraderie.

But something I wish nondisabled people understood is that being disabled isn't all doom and gloom. Yes, there are difficult parts of living in a world not built for our bodyminds. There are hardships to having to explain your existence to everyone. Some days my autocorrecting nerves get on my nerves. Yet being disabled also includes joy: laugh until you cry, side-splitting, must pause to catch your breath, abundant joy.

There's the joy of sitting above everyone else at the theater because the seat in my mobility scooter is higher than an average chair. She's giving royalty. The joy of someone's visual description including a hefty dose of sass. The joy of silent discos. The joy of sign names capturing something genuine about a person that hearing culture otherwise misses. The joy of sharing your latest disability life hack. The joy of captions as poetry. The joy of an inside joke you know only our community would laugh at, like calling myself a "roll model" or joking that "I always win at musical chairs." The joy of awe at our art.

Disabled people are some of the most joyful people I know. Perhaps it's because we've developed our own ways of being together. Perhaps it's because we know we don't have to be quiet, extraordinary, or "normal" all at the same time. Perhaps it's because we know that laughter keeps others' fear from defeating us. Joy robs ableism of its power. We know that humor reduces stress, strengthens our immune systems, releases endorphins, and relaxes our bodyminds. Laughter really is the best medicine.

Maybe that's why I have taught myself to joke and jest. Whenever someone accuses me of joking as a coping mechanism, I want to give them a gold star for being Captain Obvious. Of course I joke to cope! I use humor to put nondisabled people at ease. Nondisabled people are typically uncomfortable with my disabled bodymind, and a little joke goes a long way. Jokes cloak people's fears. Plus, it's often a delicious surprise for nondisabled people that we can be funny. Surprise, she's got jokes!

But it's much more than putting people at ease for ease's sake. I do this to resist the notion that disabled lives are not worth living. There is something disarming in a joke; it allows us to break social barriers and build a shared culture together. Jokes are a way of educating people about my humanity without condescending or cowering in the moment. They say, "You should see the other guy!" to diffuse the invasive questions about my bodymind. They ask someone to reconsider the predominant narrative about disability as tragic. They allow me to keep my dignity intact. If you're the first one to the punch line, *you* are not the punch line.

Jokes are my way of creating a shared experience. Taking charge of the moment, my jokes set a boundary for what we can laugh at together. Spoiler: It's not my disability. Jokes allow people in on aspects of my life with humor and humility instead of pestering them with facts and stats. Jokes are a form of community-building, one laugh at a time. Disabled joy is a tough pill for some to swallow. And my survival depends on other people taking that medicine.

Take, for example, when a stranger asks me, "What's wrong with you?" I can respond with a lecture or a liturgy, or I can share a laugh. Usually, I list a bunch of things that I am dealing with: (1) harping on a fellow driver honking at me for daring to let pedestrians cross the road, (2) heaping my irritation onto the two-factor authentication system just to check my email, and (3) homing in on my worst self. Turn that frown upside down by cajoling jerks into jokes. Listing instead of leering in the face of ableism. Laughing instead of lecturing.

When a stranger asks me, "Why do you use that thing?!" my go-to clapback is, "Why don't *you*?" It has a 98 percent success rate of getting their attention and bends and snaps their ableist nonsense. Or when a stranger asks, "Can I pray for you?" I reply, "Yes, but only if I can pray for you first!" If they let me, I ask God to heal their ableism. Works every time.

All of these retorts allow me to avoid the trauma dump or becoming a grump. All of these jokes are so I am not a jerk. All of these wisecracks are firmly rooted in the disability wisdom that my life is worth living and that life is radically joyful if we let it be.

Whenever joy is left out of the conversation, we are entrenched in the ableist nonsense of thinking that disabled people are slacking or lacking. That everything about disability has to be super pious or proper. Or worse, tragic. Maybe that's why nondisabled people tend to underestimate disabled people's quality of life.[4] Or why strangers chide me to cut the quips and get real. Maybe that's why so many Christians can't take a joke. We know that joy is the fruit of the Spirit, and yet all too often Christians are super serious and judgy about all the things. We are so often outraged but at all the wrong things. It's like we've forgotten there is "a time to laugh" (Eccles. 3:4).

By joy, I don't mean that we all need to be happy clappy. I think happiness is linked to external factors or fleeting moments. It's a vanishing act. But joy isn't a fickle friend. Lament and joy are not contradictions but companions. Joy is a state of being with purpose and meaning. It does not erase or pretend. My joy is not naive but nuanced. Disabled joy is an act of resistance that boldly declares that we are worthy of love and community just as we are. Part of me feels a little skeptical when someone claims that joy is a resistance just to get a mani-pedi or to excuse their inaction in the face of injustice. When I say disabled joy is resistance, I don't mean pampering or placating, I mean pushing back on the predominant narrative that disabled lives aren't worth living. My

4. National Council on Disability, "Quality-Adjusted Life Years and the Devaluation of Life with a Disability," November 6, 2019, https://www.ncd.gov/report/quality-adjusted-life-years-and-the-devaluation-of-life-with-a-disability.

joy enables strategic code-switching that sets a clear boundary of engagement and invites people into my world. It also keeps me humble. Thou shalt not be a jerk. Disabled joy declares that we are not just enough, we are exuberant. I think we need to reclaim our joy in places that people have come to least expect.

Perhaps recapturing joy is part of what Jesus meant when coaching disciples to become like children to enter the kingdom of heaven (Matt. 18:3). Children often laugh and play without much of the pretentiousness we accumulate in adulthood. Children are often not as self-conscious about their "brand" or the way they land but remain present in the moment with all its emotional roller coasters. Cue the tears and fears. Children can lead us in their joy.

Something I have learned from the embodied wisdom of children is the way they think mobility aids are marvelous. My nieces and nephews love Diana. If they had their way, they would take turns doing wheelies with her around the room. It means a lot to me that they think Diana is not defeated but dynamic.

I noticed this when I visited my niece and nephew's soccer game. To call it "soccer" is generous. Picture a gaggle of first graders reminded which way to run across the field. Goals were not the goal; community was.

Cheering from the sidelines, I overheard my nephew tell his friend, "That's my aunt. She doesn't have to walk. She gets to use a scooter!" He beamed with pride at sharing this disability wisdom with his friend. That'll preach. These two seven-year-olds could teach the church a lot about how to think about disability. They instinctively recognized the joy of disability and thought it was something exciting, not embarrassing. They didn't participate in the way we often construct hierarchies of humanity, and instead developed their own understanding of the joy that the diversity of creation can bring. They are real ones. Their joy can lead the way in people unlearning some of the lies we've been told about disability as deficit, and usher in a new way of understanding us as divine. Let their joy guide us to co-create a new way of being together.

Joy is a holistic rewiring. It carves out space in our neuropathways to dream that another world is possible. Joy is not just a fleeting feeling. Joy is an embodiment, a practice, a way of moving through the world. In my experience, reverence, gratitude, and grief can be gateways to joy. It is neither naive nor escapist like its capricious cousin, bliss. Joy makes us believe that an abundant life is possible. I am not talking about having a lot of stuff or any other traps of materialism. (I'm told I am a minimalist.) I am talking about the embodied experience of knowing that we have enough and we are enough. Joy is pivotal in the journey to justice.

Disabled people have long developed cultural practices that celebrate our access needs as invitations to cultivate joy and build community. Look no further than a visual description to provide access for anyone who is blind or low vision. The idea is to share any visible attributes that might be helpful for someone to know. Mine usually goes a little something like this: "I am a disabled, white Australian woman wearing a dinosaur dress so you think I am fun. I am sitting in my mobility scooter, bedazzled with a *W* for Wonder Woman, so you remember who you're talking to."

My visual description isn't about title, it's about testimony. It's about me—dinosaur-wearing, bedazzled me—who would like to think of myself as Wonder Woman. It's an invitation to know how I think about and talk about my wheels as an asset and want others to do the same.

My visual description isn't merely creating access. It's an invitation to be in community with me, to know something authentic about me. I have learned much more about friends, students, and colleagues through their visual descriptions than their appearance. It's a way to get to know what features are important to someone in their understanding of themselves. It invites a community of care. Visual descriptions can be joyful, irreverent, and sassy. They are cultural artifacts based on valuing the wholeness of a person rather than just someone's accomplishments or accolades, which are not apparent. Visual descriptions are a way of creating joyful access.

Another joyful cultural practice is sign names. Sign names are given by a Deaf person as a way of developing a shorthand for signing someone's name. Instead of repeatedly fingerspelling each letter of someone's name, we can use their sign name. For example, my friend Brandy's sign name is the *b* handshape over the face in the sign for "beautiful." What a humble brag. Her sign name means she's beautiful. Instead of fingerspelling B-R-A-N-D-Y every time someone refers to her, we use her sign name. Another friend's sign name uses the sign for "happy." Another's? The sign for "shy." A sign name can only be bestowed on someone by a Deaf person and is an important part of Deaf culture. Sign names connect with something that makes you *you*. It is a joyful practice of cultivating community in communication.

The disability community has shown me how skilled we are at creating ways of being together that use accessibility as a joyful tool for possibility-making. We do this through visual descriptions, sign names, sensory tools, and inside jokes. We know that our joy and cultural practices can help hatch a space for all of us to thrive. We know what it is to live a life outside of calendars and clocks, and that our spoons are sacred.[5] We are the face that time rejects. We are the future, living in the now, in a timeline that is not ready for us.

We know how communication can be enhanced by signing. We value the spatial awareness and intimacy that Deaf culture brings. We know the benefit of learning about someone's personality through their visual description. We know how children can teach us the merriment of mobility aids, and we want to follow their joy into a new creation. We shape community from our living

5. Kay Ulanday Barrett, "To Be Underwater and Holy," *The Deaf Poet's Society* 3 (January 2017), https://www.deafpoetssociety.com/kay-ulanday-barrett.

rooms, our beds, and our shared experiences of being forgotten. We might joke to cope and to buttress ourselves from the ableist nonsense. We move at the speed of love.[6]

All of this joy can help us understand the divine a little bit better each day. Some of us have been taught to bifurcate ourselves into what happens on Sundays and what happens the rest of the week. But there is no separation of sacred and secular when it comes to what Creator cares about. As Rachel Held Evans reminds us, "Ours is a God who knows how to mend clothes and bake bread, a God familiar with the planting and harvest seasons, the traditions of bridesmaids, and the tickle of wool on the back of the neck."[7] God is immersed in the cares of creation and deeply embedded in the lives of the beloved. The way we cook, clean, communicate, and create all matter to God. I believe our joy matters, and it matters to God. The God we meet in Scripture tells us stories, sings us songs, whispers to us, and celebrates us. Creator tells us that we messy masterpieces are *very* good. God chooses to dwell among us. God is with us.

God is not confined to the church alone.[8] God is in the surgery as much as in the sanctuary. God is in the sleeper town and the Big Apple as much as in the chapel. God is in the playhouse as much as the pulpit. And God's divine image is in disabled people.

One of the uncomfortable truths is that disabled people are often treated with more love, respect, and kindness *outside* of church walls than within. We can change that. We can co-create a world where disability is not vilified but venerated. We don't need to apologize for our existence or explain our joy. We can celebrate and radiate our disability wisdom to the world until one

6. Kosuke Koyama, *Three Mile an Hour God* (Orbis Books, 1980).

7. Rachel Held Evans, *Inspired: Slaying Giants, Walking on Water, and Loving the Bible Again* (Nelson, 2018), 161.

8. For more on how physical spaces are spiritual spaces, check out Kaitlin B. Curtice, *Native: Identity, Belonging, and Rediscovering God* (Brazos, 2020), 6–11.

day, talking about disability and joy in the same sentence won't seem suspect or even surprising.

My joy is an expression of my hope that we can create another way of being together that doesn't sneer or stare at us—any of us—but celebrates us. My joy is a forebearer of a world where disabled people are not routinely excluded but expected. My joy is a faithful witness that defies ableist nonsense in all its forms. My joy is an outflow of the hope that another world is not just possible but probable.

And until we get there, may our joy light the way, offering us a glimpse of what that world could be, one laugh at a time.

PRACTICE

Laugh. What is something that makes you laugh? Maybe it's a person, a movie, or an animal. What is something that brings you joy? Maybe it's swimming, rolling really fast down a hill, or putting on your noise-canceling headphones. What is something that you take delight in? Maybe it's dancing, doodling, or dessert.

Whatever it is, make a plan to find a moment of joy today. What we focus on grows. It doesn't have to be grand or gigantic. It can be a chuckle at an inside joke between friends, a moment of connection over boba, or showing up for someone who needs it. If you can, try not to shame yourself for it. Our pleasure doesn't have to be guilty. Joy doesn't have to be earned or burned. It can be shared.

ACKNOWLEDGMENTS

This book was written in the in between: in between meetings with students and colleagues, in between DCC events, in between doctor's appointments, hospital stints, and medical procedures, and in between phases when it was too painful to leave bed. I think of this book less as the thoughts of an individual and more as an overflow of the wonderful and wacky communities I am honored to call my own. I am grateful to be surrounded by a community of friends and (chosen) family who have nourished my soul and life in ways too numerous to recount here. If you have been a part of any of these communities, I thank you for the role you played, even if you are not mentioned here by name.

Thank you to Katelyn Beaty, Erin Smith, Eric Salo, and the Brazos team for being excited about this book. To the people who generously read chapters and offered gracious feedback: Brenna Jones, Erin Arendse, Julia Watts Belser, Erna Kim Hackett, Brandi Miller, Kevin Nye, Fr. Greg Schenden, DIRECTOR Rev. Ebony Grisom, Jermaine Jones, Emily Mendenhall, Annie Selak, and Chanté Griffin, I am grateful for your kind, witty, and insightful comments that improved this book. I am even more grateful to get to be in community with each of you.

To my radiant disability community, I am so thankful to be among you. Julia Watts Belser, thank you for your wonderful disability kinship that has encouraged me to love crows. Alice Sheppard, thank you for your disability wisdom on and off the stage, especially in our rich conversations. Thank you to our Disability ERG, Lachi, Ly Xīnzhèn M. Zhǎngsūn Brown, Maria Town, Douglas Kearney, Laurel Lawson, Colin Clark, Tatiana Cholewa, Sara M. Acevedo, Margaret Fink, Dani Lucchese, Christine Sun Kim, Alice Wong, Lacey Lescault, Jenny Cavallero, Kat Williams, Ren Lescault, and Tiffany Meehan for your work, joy, rage, and rest in support of our community.

Thank you to Kelly Otter and Darryl Christmon for believing in me more than I believe in myself. Thank you to Amanda Phillips for not forgetting that we are real. Thank you to my colleagues for cheering me on, who are too many to name here and include Kernysha Rowe, Bill Cessato for "Who's Amy?" delight, Lionell Daggs III, Carolyn Forché, Aminatta Forna, Andria Wisler, Stanley Bahorek, Charlene Brown-Mckenzie, Madeline Vitek Memenza, Joel Michael Reynolds, Anupam Chakravarty, Bisi Okubadejo, Rachel Kohli, Justin Smith, Antonio Lyons, Rabia Shinaishin, Kim Mazyck, Javier Jiménez Westerman, and many more. Thank you to our students, who I am privileged to get to work with every day in creating a world where we can all co-flourish.

On a more personal note, thank you to my sister for the happy hours, to my "Born in the 80s" group chat, and to my family for being excited about this book. All my gratitude to Ruth for your continued partnership in making "three friends and a dream" a Jubilee Homes reality. Brenna, thank you for being the sick light of the hurricane's eye. May the stars always align for us to spontaneously meet in an elevator on the 29th floor. Erin, thank you for being the screaming hawk. May we always find ways to meet in Seattle for biscuits and community.

And to Andrew, who has kept me fueled with honey-halva mochas, encouraging advice, and ample amounts of laughter at even my most mundane puns: My life is more joyful and vibrant with you in it. I always want to wave from such great heights with you.

AMY KENNY (PhD) is a disabled scholar-practitioner and the founding director of the Disability Cultural Center at Georgetown University, one of only a handful of such centers in the country. She is the award-winning author of *My Body Is Not a Prayer Request*, and her work on disability has appeared in *Teen Vogue*, *Sojourners*, *HuffPost*, *Reader's Digest*, and *Shondaland*. She also cofounded Jubilee Homes, a housing initiative for people experiencing homelessness.

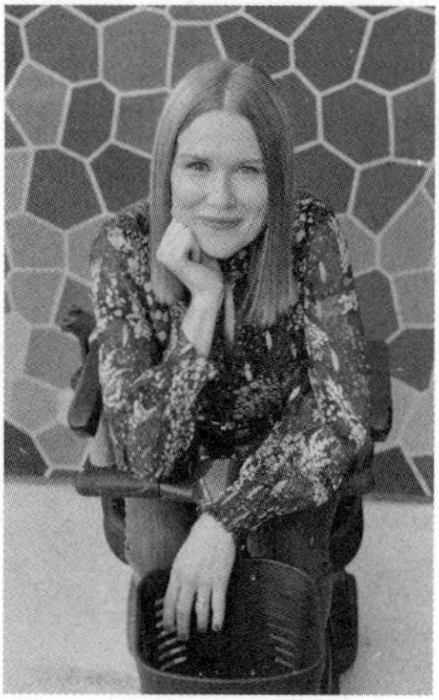

To access a Spotify playlist of songs intended to accompany this book, scan the code below: